The Empathic Practitioner

Empathy, Gender, and Medicine

EDITED BY ELLEN SINGER MORE
AND MAUREEN A. MILLIGAN

Rutgers University Press
New Brunswick, New Jersey

Library of Congress Cataloging-in-Publication Data

The Empathic practitioner : empathy, gender, and medicine /
  edited by Ellen Singer More and Maureen A. Milligan.
    p.   cm.
  Includes bibliographical references and index
  ISBN 0–8135–2118–1 (cloth) — ISBN 0–8135–2119–X (pbk.)
  1. Physician and patient. 2. Empathy. 3. Women physicians.
I. More, Ellen Singer, 1946– . II Milligan, Maureen A., 1958–
  [DNLM: 1. Empathy. 2. Physician-Patient Relations. 3. Sex
Factors. BF 575.E55 E548 1994]
R727.3.E477 1994
610.69'6—dc20
DNLM/DLC
for Library of Congress   94-10061
                                                   CIP

British Cataloging-in-Publication information available

Contents

Section One / Empathy and the Profession of Medicine

Section Two / Empathy, Ambiguity, and the Problem of Professional Authority

Section Three / Managing Vulnerability: Power, Empowerment, and Empathy in the Clinical Setting

Section Four / Empathy and the Politics of Difference

Acknowledgments

Volume editors are generally thought to need the patience of Job and the politics of Gandhi—or so the stories suggest. Our experience was different. Both of us are grateful for the experience of a genuinely stimulating and productive collaboration. But this volume is the result of the commitment, cooperation, and support of many individuals, especially our contributors. These we wish to thank first. We also wish to acknowledge Ron Carson and the University of Texas Medical Branch's Institute for the Medical Humanities for generous support for and encouragement of the original idea of an interdisciplinary conference on empathy and gender. Our Institute colleagues, as always, provided just the right combination of enthusiasm and skepticism throughout this project. We are also indebted to Joan Phillips, Eleanor Porter, and especially Dorothy Karilanovic for their excellent editorial and secretarial assistance. Maureen Milligan wishes to thank Professor David Cordova and the Division of Health Care Administration at UTMB for supporting her work at the Institute. Ellen More wishes to thank Marlie Wasserman, formerly of Rutgers University Press, for enthusiastic support and savvy editorial advice. The editors Marilyn Campbell and Karen Reeds and copyeditor Elizabeth Gretz all provided highly professional assistance. To the close friends who gave crucial support at the critical moments, we will always be grateful. Finally, Ellen More wishes to thank Elizabeth More—a more empathic daughter would be hard to imagine.

The Empathic Practitioner

MAUREEN A. MILLIGAN AND
ELLEN SINGER MORE

Introduction

Fred Astaire: What's empathicalism?

Audrey Hepburn: It's the most sensible approach to true understanding and peace of mind.

Astaire: But what is it?

Hepburn: It's based on empathy. Do you know what *empathy* means?

Astaire: No, I'll have to have the beginner's course on that one. Empathy . . . is it something like *sympathy*?

Hepburn: Oh, it goes beyond sympathy. Sympathy is to understand what someone feels. Empathy is to project your imagination so that you actually feel what the other person is feeling. You put yourself in the other person's place. Do I make myself clear?

[Astaire kisses Hepburn and she, outraged, demands to know why.]

Astaire: Empathy. I put myself in your place and felt you wanted to be kissed.

Hepburn: You were in the *wrong* place.

Scene from *Funny Face* (1957)

As patients, many of us have felt a bit like Audrey Hepburn. Our doctors are either in the "wrong place" or they don't seem to be "there" at all. Practitioners and patients often have the feeling that they just do not connect. But why not? What factors prevent any of us, but particularly physicians, from being empathic? Professional training? Time constraints? Fear of intimacy? Or the (mistaken) belief that empathy is irrelevant to good health care: a luxury at best, a dangerous distraction at worst?[1] To be sure, many physicians provide empathic care to their patients; yet many others express a genuine ambivalence toward empathy. What contribution can empathy make to modern health care and medicine?

Take, for example, the experience of Mrs. J and her seventeen-year-old daughter, Karen. Since birth Karen had experienced motor difficulties, a severe seizure disorder, an inability to speak, and mental retardation. She was, however, able to enjoy life and to bring joy into the lives of others. Karen enjoyed food, music, swimming, and her cat, Henry. She went to school, knew how to sign, and could communicate fully with her mother and father. Her parents did not see her as "sick."

She was Karen. Mrs. J recounted taking Karen for her semiannual visit to her neurologist. He examined her as he had done at least twice a year for the past fifteen years. After the examination, he noticed Karen signing to her mother. Startled, he commented that Karen "*does* know what is going on." For all his work with Karen's brain, the physician did not know Karen—the depth of her relationship with her parents and her capacity for enjoyment, understanding, communication, and relationships. Did his failure to understand much of his patient's inner experience affect his relationship with Karen? Did it affect the quality of the care he gave her? Mrs. J's deep anger signs to us that it did.[2]

Karen's story illustrates important truths about how physicians have been trained to approach the patient-physician relationship, the "ways of knowing" that characterize those relationships in modern medicine, and their implications for empathic communication. Medicine's modern adaptation to the culture of science has had serious implications for the ethical core of clinical medicine: the therapeutic relationship. As many historians have argued, it has produced a profound change in the professional identity of American physicians. Prior to the late nineteenth century, medical practice was grounded explicitly in a deep familiarity not only with the physical but also with the psychological, spiritual, and social particularities of patients, their families, and their communities. Dominant medical theory presumed that these variables significantly affected the course of health and disease. An intimate understanding of these factors was therefore thought to be crucial for good care.

Changes in medicine's theoretical orientation and the subsequent restructuring of health care institutions gradually reordered diagnostic and therapeutic priorities. The theoretical grounding of practice shifted from a personal knowledge of unique individuals to the universal and objective knowledge of physiological processes. The traditional importance of interpersonal knowledge and skills was gradually eclipsed by values of objectivity, quantification, universality, and control. John Harley Warner has noted that the "experimental therapeutist's attention was closely centered on a physiological process rather than an individual patient, and in some respects it made relatively little difference whether that process was going on in an Irish immigrant or a laboratory dog."[3] New criteria for what would count as knowledge gave direction to medical research as well as to clinical practice. The narrowness of the criteria, however, excluded important—albeit ambiguous—types of knowledge: interpersonal knowledge that could not easily be quantified, controlled, or explained. With the development and increasing use of sophisticated diagnostic techniques, objective quantifiable data *displaced* patients' subjective reports of symptoms. Karen's experience suggests that these changes can minimize both the patient's active role in his or her own care and the perceived importance of patient-physician relationships for the acquisition and interpretation of diagnostic data.[4]

A century and a half after the beginnings of medicine's bacteriological revolution, physicians are still seeking to reconcile "scientific" styles of thought and practice with the interpersonal skills so central to successful healing. The stress on "scientific" objectivity—the physician as diagnostician, the patient as "object of study"—has not made this an easy task. Modern medicine's stringent epistemological standards often constrain the possibility of empathic practice.

While medicine seeks certainty and control, empathy requires vulnerability and humility. Our capacity to know other persons may be limited, ambiguous, and uncertain, yet it is also incredibly powerful. Empathy requires a willingness and an ability to leave the security of one's own beliefs, feelings, and frame of reference at least briefly in order to approach the feelings, thoughts, and world of another. This "back and forth" movement between self and other is captured in the definition of empathy given by Alexandra Kaplan, a psychologist at the Stone Center for Developmental Services and Studies at Wellesley College. Empathy, she writes, is "the capacity to take in and appreciate the affective life of another while maintaining a sufficient sense of self to permit cognitive structuring of that experience."[5] The cognitive, affective, and psychological requirements of empathy make it a challenging and rewarding part of any interpersonal relationship.

Recent discussions of empathy, generated within the growing field of medical humanities, consider it integral not just to psychiatry but to all aspects of clinical medicine.[6] Yet medicine's standards of what counts as knowledge, and its goals of objectivity, certainty, and control (or avoidance) of emotion, make the practice of empathic medicine particularly challenging.[7] Not only have epistemological and professional standards discouraged development of empathic practices, the patients and families with whom one connects in health care settings often manifest profound needs, fears, and deep physical, emotional, and/or existential suffering. Fear of the suffering experienced by many patients presents many care givers with a formidable barrier to the empathic practice of medicine. Some providers recoil, consciously or unconsciously, from the possibility of sharing this suffering and vulnerability.

In our discussions of empathy with students and clinicians of all sorts, the objection we most frequently encounter arises from the fear that the practice of empathic expertise will exhaust, not regenerate, the spirit. Fear of losing control, of the depleting effects of unguarded openness to one's patients, is a persistent theme in the literature on empathy.[8] One physician acknowledged, "I am aware of how draining and threatening empathy for helpless, injured people can be."[9]

Certainly, under any circumstances, empathy is neither an easy nor a straightforward process. Particularly within a culture like medicine, blurring the distance between one's patient and oneself—even momentarily—would seem to invite diagnostic and therapeutic chaos. Perri Klass writes: "The nitty-gritty detail of being a doctor requires a certain amount of detachment. You cannot put down a nasogastric tube if you are imagining too graphically the passage of that tube into your own throat."[10] Empathic practice requires the negotiation of a practical balance between connection with another and the maintenance of one's sense of self. It is often accomplished through an alliance of technical skill and interpersonal attunement, through the self-conscious, ethical choice to enter into the inner world of the patient. Ideally, this balanced practice of empathy in the therapeutic relationship, in Lucy Candib's words, makes possible the "readiness to feel the other's feelings as one's own and to use that awareness for the benefit of the other."[11]

We therefore believe that any ethical practice of medicine requires a certain amount of empathy. Beneficence and respect are among the oldest principles of medical ethics. To what degree can patients' best interests be advanced if care givers know relatively little about the patient, his or her world, values, or interests? According to the philosopher Iris Marion Young, "justice begins in a hearing, in heeding a call, rather than in asserting and mastering a state of affairs."[12] We believe that empathy, like justice, is a kind of listening, first to the "other" (the patient), then to oneself, then to the patient again. We "do justice" to patients by engaging in the attempt to act fittingly toward them. *Complete* understanding cannot be our standard of empathic practice, for that is virtually never within our grasp. Empathy need not—we believe it cannot—be perfect; but it can—and must—represent a good faith effort to "hear" the other.

In the early 1960s Robert Katz wrote of the therapeutic and ethical importance of empathic professionalism: "The mark of a good empathizer is the respect [s/]he has for the integrity of his [or her] client."[13] Katz believes that people need to feel that someone else "not only understands our words but appreciates the person behind the message as well. We then know that we are recognized and accepted for the particular kind of person we are. . . . When empathy is lacking, our self-awareness and self-respect are diminished. We then experience ourselves more as objects and less as persons." As growing evidence from psychoneuroimmunology suggests, care givers who assist the healing process by truly paying heed to their patients and respecting their integrity enhance (rather than hamper) their technical skill.[14]

It is equally important, we believe, to acknowledge and respect the practitioner's own need for integrity. The tension between public and personal identity implicit in the very idea of "professionalism" has proved profoundly detrimental to many practitioners' sense of personal integration and responsibility. In its desire to shun the subjective and personal in favor of the objective and universal, scientific professionalism risks detaching personal responsibility from technical expertise. Professionals who are in a real sense *personally* absent from their patients miss essential detail by remaining at a distance. We argue that this distanced "professional" stance also undermines physicians' ability to be fair, fitting, and optimally effective in their practice. We are unconvinced by claims that adopting a stance of neutrality or "objectivity" toward patients will minimize diagnostic and therapeutic errors or the prejudicial effects of race, gender, and social class. More often, such "objectivity" obscures recognition of the patient as person and hides the effects of prejudice (whether about gender, class, race, or ethnicity). In the long run, attempts to bridge such distances and differences make for better medicine than retreating to a distanced objectivity.[15] Overcoming these distances also provides the sense of connection with patients that is typically a source of deep satisfaction and fulfillment for most physicians.

Nevertheless, we realize the significant dangers associated with empathy. Therapeutic "knowing" can turn into imperial intrusion. Rather than giving patients their "voice," the act of "empathic imagination," as Alfred Margulies puts it, may put our words and thoughts into their mouths.[16] Susan Griffin writes in *A Chorus of Stones,* "It is a delicate balance, telling someone else's story, entering another life, identifying, feeling as this other might have felt, and yet remaining aware that a boundary exists over which one cannot step."[17] Even with the best intentions it is all too easy, like Fred Astaire, to put oneself in the "wrong" place. Responsible empathic practice requires a vigilant sensitivity to the potential for harm when physicians and others engage in the intimate dance of empathic encounter.

At a 1992 conference, "Empathic Expertise: Gender, Empathy, and the Therapeutic Relationship," held at the Institute for the Medical Humanities of the University of Texas Medical Branch at Galveston, the historical, epistemological, gender, ethical, literary, and clinical implications of the role of empathy in medical care were explored by a

group of scholars from a wide range of humanistic and clinical specialties. The essays in this volume were developed from that conference
and represent our attempt to broach the relationship between empathy
and gender in the culture of modern medicine.

Although most of the essays focus on the role of physicians, we are
aware that empathy plays perhaps an even larger role in the practice of
other health care professionals. We have chosen to focus primarily on
medicine because the centrality of the scientific paradigm of objectivity
and distance makes the practice of empathy especially challenging for
physicians.

Five general concerns dominated our discussions and shaped the
goals of our inquiry: First, exactly what do we mean by the term "empathy"? How is it defined? How does it differ from sympathy? How
have its definitions evolved historically, and what does this evolution
tell us about the adaptation of empathy for the work of modern professionalism? Second, how does empathy "work"? What does it mean to
be empathic? Does it mean that one truly "knows," with certainty,
what another is feeling and thinking? How much can any one person
know of another's thoughts and feelings? Third, how empathic ought
one be—and specifically, how empathic should health care providers
be? Is empathy an asset, a responsibility, or a liability in health care?
Fourth, how do health care providers, particularly physicians, practice
empathy in clinical settings? What are the rewards, advantages, obstacles, and risks of being an empathic practitioner? Furthermore, how
do differences of culture, gender, race, social class, professional education, and values affect practitioners' ability to be empathic? Fifth, can
empathy be learned? If so, how can we encourage or train young practitioners to open themselves to the possibilities of empathic practice?
Each of the essays in this book addresses aspects of these problems—
sometimes from the perspective of the patient or practitioner, sometimes through the perspective of the historian, sometimes through
philosophy or literature.

In Section One we place the concept of "empathy" in historical context.
What historical forces impelled the introduction of empathy into the
professional discourse of medicine and gave rise to its contested meanings? The chapters by the historians Ellen S. More, Regina Morantz-
Sanchez, and Susan E. Lederer illustrate how the new values of
professionalism, in alliance with changing gender norms, affected the
patient-practitioner relationship. The concept of empathy, they emphasize, was introduced to clinical medicine amid these changes.

More argues that empathy's importation into medicine was regulated by the tensions between gender and professionalism in the late nineteenth century. She asks, "What cultural 'work' was a 'relational' concept like empathy designed to accomplish within the objectifying culture of twientieth-century medicine?" The term "empathy" first appeared in the psychology of aesthetics to signify an emotional connection between subject and object—a discursively feminine meaning that has persisted in popular definitions of empathy. It was introduced into medical theory and practice for quite different purposes. At a time when medical professionalism increasingly mimicked the values and behaviors of experimental science, physicians required an appropriate protocol by which to regulate the intimacies of the patient-physician relationship. Traditionally, the metaphor of "sympathy" had governed this relationship. More argues that during the Victorian era the connotative meaning of sympathy became feminine and sentimental, disqualifying it from professional legitimacy. In its place, especially within psychoanalysis, empathy was fashioned into a "technique for the acquisition of knowledge about the subjective experience of the patient" while maintaining the professionally mandatory interpersonal boundaries. Ultimately, empathy came to represent what More calls the "ideal mediator between comfort and risk" for all clinical medicine. By the 1960s it became a linchpin of the movement in medical education to teach what was called "detached concern." In the past two decades or so, this detachment has increasingly been perceived to be problematic. Recent feminist and postmodern emphases on interpretation and intersubjectivity have made possible a repositioning and reinterpretation of the role of empathy in medicine.

Regina Morantz-Sanchez chronicles the widening divergence between traditional and modern conceptions of the physician-patient relationship by comparing the careers of two late nineteenth-century women physicians, Elizabeth Blackwell and Mary Dixon-Jones. She highlights the differences between the older model of "sympathetic understanding" and a newer one based on the values of "objective" science. Elizabeth Blackwell's holistic approach to medical care called for "sympathetic" understanding of patients' unique histories as factors in their health and disease. Blackwell specifically framed sympathy as distinct from technical, reductionist medical science, associating the former with women and the latter with men. Mary Dixon-Jones, in contrast, displayed a very different approach to medical care. Jones strove to master surgical techniques and to gown herself in the crisp respectability of the new scientific medicine, developing a reputation in gynecological surgery and surgical pathology. She published articles in leading journals and crafted a reputation as a member of the scientific and surgical elite. Eventually charged with manslaughter and malpractice, however, Jones came to symbolize social fears that the new bacteriological model would promote insensitivity to, and abuse of, patients. Her case seemed to prove that sympathy for patients would be abandoned as medicine adopted a bacteriological reductionism and moved toward surgical solutions to disease. The gendering of sympathy as feminine and science as masculine made Jones appear even more aberrant and frightening in the subsequent court trials.

Susan Lederer uses the antivivisectionist movement to chronicle the gendered divergence between sympathy and science in the late nineteenth century. Vivisection represented both the corruption of traditional professional values and the modus operandi of the new science, and as such became the target of heated debates. Antivivisectionists were concerned that vivisection and the biologically reductionist attitude it fostered would harden medical students to their future patients just as, they claimed, it hardened them to the suffering of animals. Vivisectionists attacked antivivisectionists' efforts to interfere with research by labeling sympathy for animal welfare as "feminine," irrational, and pathologically emotional. The controversy ultimately promoted the conflation of caring in general with feminine, irrational, and overly emotional attitudes and behavior. As overt expressions of sympathy became increasingly gendered, they became more problematic for both male and female physicians. This gendering of care as "feminine" hampered attempts to incorporate the new bacteriological sciences and sympathetic care into a unified image of medical professionalism, further widening the gap between sympathy and science.

Section Two explores the epistemological and psychological roots of professional anxiety about the practice of empathy in patient-practitioner relationships. Medical science's quest for certainty and control was understandable during an era plagued with endemic diseases and illnesses, a shortened life expectancy, and none of the vaccinations or antibiotics we take for granted today. Yet as some of the authors in this section argue, the quest for certainty and control in knowledge often conceals something deeper—a fear of ambiguity, intimacy, and interdependence. Philosophers such as Susan Bordo and Jane Flax, for example, have hypothesized a connection between the epistemological quest for certainty and the psychological quest for security.[18] The second section of this book therefore considers how epistemological, psychological, and social dis-ease with ambiguity and uncertainty shaped the answer to the question of what counts as knowledge—particularly knowledge of the patient. How this knowledge is construed determines social and professional perceptions about the possibility, value, and ethical significance of empathy, issues explored in Section Three.

The philosopher Lorraine Code lays bare the theoretical threads woven into the social construction of knowledge and analyzes their impact on the epistemological and social status of empathy. Because of their allegiance to the values of universality, formalistic abstraction, certainty, control, and nonaffectivity, standard theories of knowledge interpret the notion of "empathetic knowledge" as oxymoronic; empathy *cannot* be a form of knowing. Code challenges these assumptions. The obsession with control and certitude invalidates ways of knowing essential for human life and relationships and devalues the skills necessary for these ways of knowing. Because the discourse of gender in European and American culture associates women with relational and empathic knowing, women and their skills are also devalued. Code suggests that hermeneutics might provide a theoretical grounding for empathic knowing since it can accommodate ambiguity and, therefore, knowledge about life as it is lived, without succumbing to the chaos of epistemological relativism.

Code also alerts those who would advocate the value of empathy to three specific dangers that accompany its use. First, she is leery of the essentialism underlying the claim that empathy is a "natural" female trait. Second, she is concerned that empathy will be used merely as a professional, scientific construct, belittled in women but valued as a "skill" when practiced in a professional context. Third, she is concerned that empathy could be abused in asymmetrical power relations; professionals could use claims of expertise to *tell* others "just how they feel." Code concludes by considering the ethical-political implications of empathic knowing. Citing Simone de Beauvoir's *The Ethics of Ambiguity*, she asserts that an ethics/politics that legitimates appropriate empathic knowledge could counter the dehumanizing power of bureaucracy and be more sensitive to ambiguity, individuality, particularity, and relationship.

While Code draws our attention to the dangers involved in those who would *tell* us "just how we feel," the psychiatrist Joan Lang draws our attention to a different danger associated with the power of empathy. In her analysis of empathy, Lang argues that "accurate attunement" to another—perceptions about the other's thoughts and feelings—is a process separate from the action one subsequently takes based on that knowledge. Knowledge of an individual's fears and his or her desire to please, to be accepted, to be loved can be used to control and manipulate behavior. Thus Lang points to the potential for abuse by those who are empathic, that is, who are accurately attuned, but who are not benevolent, not motivated to use their intimate knowledge for good. Lang's approach to the use of empathy grows out of her own clinical experience and the psychoanalyst Heinz Kohut's seminal work in self psychology. Kohut believed that the practice of empathy is value-neutral. Yet at the end of his life he also conceded a belief that the "mere presence of empathy . . . has also a beneficial, in a broad sense, a therapeutic effect—both in the clinical setting and in human life, in general."[19] Lang writes that Kohut emphasized the importance of empathy and of truly listening not only in psychoanalysis but in all healthy human relationships. But, observing the powerful human desire for empathy, she emphasizes that responsibility, accountability, and care are foundational for trust in empathic relationships.

Janet Surrey, a psychologist, and Stephen Bergman, a psychiatrist and novelist, build on the "self-with-other" relational theories developed at the Stone Center at Wellesley to argue that differences in the early psychological socialization of males and females in Western culture affect the development of empathy. They believe that the capacity for empathy is learned in relationship, that it involves cognitive and affective skills, and that women learn to be empathic in relationships with their mothers, specifically through the experience of identifying with them. Males, they argue, tend to develop "relational dread." They are encouraged to dis-identify with their mothers and to disconnect, not only from relationship with them, but from a relational "way of being" in general. Boys are taught to become "agents of disconnection." Surrey and Bergman theorize that the psychosocial structure of medical education is similar to the developmental patterns of becoming a male, and argue that the psychosocial conditions that hinder males in developing empathic relationships are reenacted during the medical education process. Using findings from their research, they identify several central impasses to mutual empathy in male-female and doctor-patient relationships. They then provide suggestions for breaking through these impasses to develop mutually empathic, empowering, authentic relationships.

As Code, Lang, and Surrey and Bergman illustrate, empathy is an epistemologically and emotionally ambiguous practice. The contributors in Section Three—all clinicians—consider from the practitioner's point of view the challenges of charting a course of empathic care. In this section Lucy Candib, Perri Klass, and Julia Connelly share how they and other physicians experience and manage vulnerability and empathy in their medical practices—how they balance connection and self-protection, power and empowerment.

Lucy Candib, a family practitioner, expands the discussion of empathy by focusing on empathy as a means to empower patients, as a prerequisite for empowerment. She outlines practices and attitudes that contribute to empowerment in clinical relationships, paying particular attention to the special concerns and needs of socially subjugated groups, especially women, the poor, and some communities of color. Respecting patients, recognizing oppression, helping patients to risk discussion of emotional needs, and legitimating patients' choices and personal power are among the practices that contribute to empathic empowerment. By using specific questions such as "How do you hope that I can help you?" and "What do you yourself think is the reason for your problem?" physicians can actively empower patients by recognizing their own wisdom, experiences, wants, and needs.

As both a pediatrician and a novelist, Perri Klass grapples with the fundamental concerns of those practitioners who would be empathic: fear of vulnerability, of pain, of overinvolvement. Physicians who practice empathic medicine strive to identify with their patients without losing their own identities as competent professionals. Identification with patients may appear to promote empathy, yet the realization that "what is happening to you could be happening to me" can propel physicians into a protective and nonempathic stance. Using the case of an infant who may (or may not) have spinal meningitis, Klass considers analogies between physicians and authors. She suggests that physicians, like authors, can be closely involved with and knowledgeable about their patients while maintaining their own identities. Like authors, they accomplish this differentiation by constructing characters: the "doctor as doctor" and the "patient as patient." In the doctor-patient relationship, both ultimately become authors of a text that narrates their common understanding of the illness.

For the internist Julia Connelly, the ability to listen is the key to engaging in successful empathic relationships. Connelly evokes in the reader a rich sense of her presence as a listener, stylistically reinforcing her message of the therapeutic power of listening—of "heeding a call." She intertwines theories of listening with personal examples, sharing her experiences of the risks and rewards of being open to patients' stories—as a medical student, as a teacher, and as a skilled practitioner. She distinguishes between what Michael Balint calls "great detective" listening and empathic listening. The first focuses on the mystery of the disease; the second also strives to understand the patient's experience. In Connelly's experience, listening to patients' experiences rather than rushing headlong into "great detective" listening not only improves the quality of the patient-physician encounter but often also improves the quality of the diagnosis. Connelly considers the relationship between listening and other aspects of the patient-physician relationship, such as control, vulnerability, and gender. She concludes with reflections on the need to promote the capacity for empathic listening in medical school.

Section Four, "Empathy and the Politics of Difference," pursues the interconnection between politics and therapeutics by examining the effects of social class, gender, and race on the practice of empathy. In varying ways the authors of these essays address the role of empathy in overcoming the tensions between the claims of "equality" and "difference" within the context of health care.[20] The psychiatrist Carol Nadelson extends Candib's analysis of empowerment by considering empathy and power in the sociopolitical realm. She develops the notion of "societal empathy" and concludes that the socio-political-economic structures of health care are not socially empathic. That is, they fail to understand the experiences of, and consequences for, those who are affected by health care policies and structures. This is due in part to the fact that many policymakers find it difficult to understand, to be empathic with, and therefore adequately to represent those who are different from themselves. Nadelson considers the ways in which bureaucracies inhibit the practice of empathy in health care, focusing on a story of one young physician's experience with managed care and on Oregon's attempts to identify objective standards for health care allocation.

Rita Charon, a general internist, and co-contributors Michele Green and Ronald Adelman, a gerontologist and an internist respectively, examine how physician gender affects the patient-physician relationship. Based on their study of patient-physician encounters, they argue that the gender of the physician affects the ways in which the physician "reads" the patient's "narrative." These different "readings" affect patient-physician communication as assessed by physician attentiveness, supportiveness, information-giving, time spent with patients, and the frequency of engaging in joint decision making. Although they note that the small sample size of the study justifies only limited generalizations from their findings, this study and its integration of narrative and feminist reader-response theories nonetheless presents a helpful model and initial empirical support for the intuitive sense that physician gender does affect the quality and likelihood of empathy in physician-patient relationships.

If, as Klass and others have suggested, empathy is aided by the capacity to understand and imaginatively enter the world of the "other," then African American women, sensitive to both gender and race oppression, may have a unique and powerful capacity for empathic exchange. Marian Gray Secundy, a medical ethicist and social worker, explores this possibility by listening to the stories of nine African American female physicians and weaving them into a narrative tapestry rich with the textures, hues, and traditions of African American females' experiences in healing. Secundy sees some historical continuity between traditional black midwives and healers and the nine physicians she interviewed. Commitment to their common heritage, the desire to be of service to others, to give of their own gifts for healing, to draw on spiritual strengths and traditions, and the capacity to understand their patients' experiences are common threads in these narratives. The physicians with whom Secundy spoke also shared a heightened awareness of the impact of socioeconomic and structural factors on the practice of their healing, for example, issues of rationing and access to care. Secundy explores how African American female physicians might differ from both their male and their white female colleagues in their medical practice and their capacity to be empathic. In a call for further study to explore these questions among a wider circle of respondents, Secundy suggests that these physicians' African American heritage may have a more profound impact than their gender on the ways they practice medicine, though both affect the patterns of their work.

Issues of difference also challenge women medical students. Exploring difference without falling prey to the dangers of essentialism presents difficult challenges. Although women generally want to leave behind the harmful stereotypes of difference ("women can't do science"), significant numbers of women medical students do express needs, perceptions, and experiences that differ from those of their male counterparts. Janet Bickel culls recent studies and her own experiences directing the Programs for Women in Medicine at the Association of American Medical Colleges to highlight those aspects of women medical students' experiences that differ from men's. These differences have implications for women's medical education and, ultimately, for the nature of their practices. Just as important, these differences serve as a basis for identifying the harmful consequences of certain aspects of traditional medical training for female *and* for male students, and therefore underscore the need to challenge some of the traditional structures and methods of medical training. In support of the work by Surrey and Bergman, Bickel notes that female students are more likely to associate isolation with danger, whereas men are more likely to identify intimacy with danger. Women medical students tend to have fewer faculty role models, have more perceived incidents of sexual harassment in medical school, and are subjected to closer scrutiny of their commitment to medicine, their spousal support, and their family plans. They also experience more role conflicts than male students. Bickel concludes her chapter with a consideration of several medical school initiatives designed to address differences and to change medical traditions, structures, and practices that equate difference with inequality.

If one theme can be said to unify so diverse a collection of essays, it is that the idea of empathy itself conceals several contested meanings within the discourse of medicine. We believe that gender has played a fundamental role in shaping these several meanings. With many differing voices, and a diversity of approaches, this book explores the ways that gender shapes both the professional discourse of medicine and the meanings imputed to the practice of empathy within the profession. It is our hope that modern medicine, through renewed attention to empathic practice, can reintegrate the essentially personal relationship that was for so long the foundation of all good practice. As these essays demonstrate, this is no simple matter, but it is essential. We hope this volume will occasion further exploration and additional dialogue.

Notes

We thank Professor Rima Apple for the reference to the epigraph.

1. Ralph R. Greenson, "Empathy and Its Vicissitudes," *Intl. J. Psycho.* 41 (1960): 418–424, esp. 418.

2. Adapted with permission from a presentation by Ellen Berman at the Institute for the Medical Humanities, University of Texas Medical Branch, Galveston, Texas, February 9, 1993.

3. John Harley Warner, *The Therapeutic Perspective* (Cambridge, Mass.: Harvard University Press, 1986), 249.

4. Cf. Stanley Joel Reiser, *Medicine and the Reign of Technology* (Cambridge: Cambridge University Press, 1978), the pioneering work on these developments.

5. Alexandra G. Kaplan, "Male or Female Psychotherapists for Women: New Formulations," in *Women's Growth in Connection: Writings from the Stone Center*, ed. Judith V. Jordan, Alexandra G. Kaplan et al. (New York: Guilford Press, 1991), 268–282.

6. James E. Rosenberg and Bernard Towers, "The Practice of Empathy as a Prerequisite for Informed Consent," *Theoretical Medicine* 7 (1987): 81–194; Howard Spiro, "What Is Empathy and Can It Be Taught?" *Ann. Int. Med.* 116: 10 (1992): 843–846; S. D. Nightingale, P. R. Yarnold, and M. S. Greenberg, "Sympathy, Empathy, and Physician Resource Utilization," *J. Gen. Int. Med.* 6 (1991): 420–423; Stanley W. Jackson, "The Listening Healer in the History of Psychological Healing," *Amer. J. Psych.* 149: 12 (December 1982): 1623–1632.

7. See the essay by Lorraine Code in this volume.

8. See the essay by Ellen More in this volume.

9. Judith Alexander Brice, "Empathy Lost," *Harvard Medical Alumni Bulletin* 60: 4 (Winter 1986–87): 28–32; cf. Charles D. Aring, "Sympathy and Empathy," *JAMA* 167: 4 (1958): 448–442.

10. See the essay by Perri Klass in this volume, 157.

11. See the essay by Lucy Candib in this volume, 138.

12. Iris Marion Young, *Justice and the Politics of Difference* (Princeton: Princeton University Press, 1990), 4. She refers here to the ideas of philosopher Jean-François Lyotard.

13. Robert L. Katz, *Empathy: Its Nature and Uses* (London: Free Press of Glencoe/Collier-Macmillan, 1963), 7, 8, 144.

14. Robert Ader, David Felten, and Nicholas Cohen, eds., *Psychoneuroimmunology*, 2nd ed. (New York: Academic Press, 1991).

15. For a discussion by an anthropologist-psychiatrist of the art of "bearing witness" to the illness narratives of patients, see Arthur Kleinman, *The Illness Narratives* (New York: Basic Books, 1988).

16. Alfred Margulies, *The Empathic Imagination* (New York: W. W. Norton and Co., 1989). E.M. is indebted to Stanley Jackson, M.D., for bringing this work to her attention.

17. Quoted in a review by Richard Restak, *New York Times Book Review*, November 22, 1992, 15.

18. Susan Bordo, *The Flight to Objectivity: Essays in Cartesianism and Culture* (Albany: State University of New York Press, 1987); Jane Flax, "Political Philosophy and the Patriarchal Unconsciousness: A Psychoanalytic Perspective on Epistemology and Metaphysics," in *Discovering Reality*, ed. Sandra Harding and Merrill Hintikka (Dordrecht: Reidel Publishing, 1983), 245–281.

19. See Joan Lang, "Is Empathy Always 'Nice'?" in this volume.

20. See Martha Minow, *Making All the Difference: Inclusion, Exclusion, and the American Law* (Ithaca, NY: Cornell University Press, 1990), for a full exposition of the "equality versus difference" dichotomy.

SECTION ONE

Empathy and the Profession of Medicine

"Empathy" Enters the Profession of Medicine

What were the pathways by which the term "empathy" first entered the profession of medicine? This essay explores the contested meanings empathy has acquired during the past century, and the role of gender in shaping those meanings.

The term "empathy" was introduced in the late nineteenth century as part of the psychology of aesthetics. Soon after, Freud adapted it to the needs of psychoanalysis.[1] It was subsequently introduced into the literature on medical education,[2] the psychology of gender,[3] and more recently, feminism and hermeneutics.[4] Some of the recent interest in empathy is a response to today's frequently *dis*-connected doctor-patient encounters. Especially within the growing field of medical humanities, empathy is increasingly discussed not only in the context of psychiatry, its point of origin within medicine, but for its potential contribution to all aspects of clinical care.[5]

Unfortunately, as I will argue, efforts to foster empathic professionalism are often held hostage to the conflicting meanings assigned to empathy within Western culture—meanings largely shaped by constructions of gender. In popular culture the term "empathy" is associated with a set of traits frequently connoted as "feminine," especially emotional attunement and identification with the feelings of others. This popular connotation is expressed as a kind of "mystical" conception akin to "feminine" intuition, "a somewhat odd and elusive skill, a divinatory art, a sixth sense, an instinctive and primitive form of penetrating to the core of another person."[6] In contrast, those who enlist "empathy" for the professional work of medicine generally resist these "feminized" associations and instead define empathy through the language of scientific objectivity. Indeed, throughout most of the twentieth century empathy has been interpreted by many psychiatrists and medical educators as a technical, discursively male-gendered practice. It has not been employed to foster "identification," to collapse the interpersonal boundaries separating patient from practitioner. Rather its function has been to contain the professional-patient relationship within limits appropriate to the emotionally neutral, scientific enterprise of modern medicine: a form of controlled intimacy. The definition found in the *International Encyclopedia of the Social Sciences* captures this technical conception: "Empathy, or empathetic understanding, is the term currently preferred by psychotherapists to designate the process and technique whereby the therapist consciously adopts the 'internal frame of reference' of the patient without losing his own identity."[7]

For centuries, before the invention of this new term and the regulated techniques of doctor-patient communication it represented, the metaphor of "sympathy" supplied a broadly serviceable model not only for the doctor-patient relationship but for the fundamentals of human physiology and the etiology of disease. But Victorian culture steadily sentimentalized, feminized, and marginalized sympathy's connotative meaning, while at the same time the term was slowly devalued within medicine's scientific and professional discourse. By the late nineteenth century the sentimentalized, feminized, holistic metaphor of sympathy was less and less adequate to the language of medicine. When a new, technical language was needed for the relationship between patients and practitioners, the devaluation of "sympathy" disqualified it for this new task. "Empathy" in its technical sense is the linguistic artifact of these developments.

What cultural "work" was a "relational" concept like empathy designed to accomplish within the objectifying culture of twentieth-century medicine? How has the politics of gender shaped our expectations and use of the concept? In this essay I first trace the process by which sympathy became marginal to medical discourse by the turn of the century. The next section examines empathy's twentieth-century career, first as a technique of psychoanalytic data collection and, later, as part of the language of medical education under the neo-Oslerian banner of "detached concern." In the final section I consider recent discussions of empathic knowledge that assert its power to combine both affective and cognitive modalities. By releasing empathy from its artificially dichotomized construction either as a "feminine" or a "masculine" way of knowing, these recent efforts may help reinvigorate empathy's role in the clinical encounter.

Sympathy, Empathy, and the Professionalization of Medicine

Although frequently traced to the work of Sigmund Freud,[8] empathy originated within the field of aesthetics. Robert Vischer, the German philosopher of aesthetics, coined the word in 1872. Vischer was trying to understand the process by which a work of art can call forth an emotional response from the observer, a momentary fusion of subject and object. The term he chose, *Einfühlung* ("feeling-into," as contrasted with sympathy or "feeling-with"), was translated into English in 1897 as "empathic projection" by "Vernon Lee" (Violet Page) and C. Anstruther-Thompson, and as "empathy" by the psychologist E. B. Titchener in 1909.[9]

Freud was introduced to the concept through the works of the German psychologist Theodor Lipps in the 1890s. According to Freud's English translator James Strachey, Lipps's influence can be seen in Freud's 1905 work, *Jokes and Their Relation to the Unconscious*, in which he discusses the role of empathy in humor. Freud noted that when we laugh at a joke, "we take the producing person's psychical state into consideration, put ourselves into it and try to understand it by comparing it with our own." These processes of "empathy and comparison," he wrote, provoke our laughter. Significantly, in *Group Psychology and the Analysis of the Ego* (1921), Freud referred to empathy during a discussion of ego integrity, "identification," and the psychology of the group, an association that continues to characterize debate over the term.[10]

Charles Edward Gauss and, more recently, Paul Rabinow and William Sullivan identified a second vector by which the concept of empathy, if not the word itself, entered the modern critical tradition, namely, through the hermeneutical operation known as *verstehen*, or "understanding," an extension of nineteenth-century biblical interpretation that acknowledged the perspective of the interpreter, developed principally by Schleiermacher, Dilthey, and Weber. Recent philosophic and psychoanalytic studies of empathy draw parallels to hermeneutic interpretive practices in the self-consciousness, or reflexivity, that characterizes empathic knowledge.[11] A current dictionary entry defines empathy as "identification with and understanding of another's situation, feelings, and motives," a definition combining both affective and cognitive connotations ("identification" and "understanding").[12]

"Empathy" often is contrasted to "sympathy."[13] I argue that although empathy was neither derived from nor a direct replacement for the concept of sympathy, it did serve as a corrective or a supplement to it—fulfilling the promise of interpersonal resonance sought in the traditional idea of sympathy but without connoting vagueness or sentimentality. This exchange was effected through a negative shift in the cultural valence attached to the concept of "sympathy," and by gradual changes in the cultural and conceptual meaning of doctor-patient communication.[14]

The *Oxford English Dictionary* defines sympathy as "a (real or supposed) affinity between certain things, by virtue of which they are similarly or correspondingly affected by the same influence, affect or influence one another (especially in some occult way), or attract or tend towards each other." In earlier times, the concept of sympathy was invoked as a model for the operation of the nervous system (a "rapport" effected throughout the body by the operation of the nerves).[15] The metaphor of "sympathy" also helped structure the meaning of doctor-patient relationships, signifying the broadly contextual knowledge of the patient believed essential to good diagnosis and therapeutics. The Edinburgh physician John Gregory, for example, believed that sympathy was the chief moral quality of the humane physician. "Sympathy," he wrote, "produces an anxious attention to a thousand little circumstances that may tend to relieve the patient." Thus by the eighteenth century the term was commonly used in both physiological and psychological senses: "the consent of one part with another, or a fellow-feeling of the same passion."[16]

Sympathy also contributed to the language of moral philosophy and politics. John Locke and other Enlightenment philosophers understood it as vital to the capacity for moral reasoning. Lockean sensationalism presumed all persons to have been born into a common state of natural equality that made possible the capacity for sympathy (or "fellow feeling") and moral sentiment.[17] David Hume, like Locke and Francis Hutcheson before him, described sympathy as a "contagion" or susceptibility. "As in strings equally wound up," Hume wrote, "the motion of one communicates itself to the rest; so all the affections readily pass from one person to another, and beget correspondent movements in every human creature.... No passion of another discovers itself immediately to the mind. We are only sensible of its causes or effects. From *these* we infer the passion; and consequently *these* [observable causes or effects] give rise to our sympathy."[18] Drawing out the implications of Humean psychology (and foreshadowing usage of the term "empathy"), Adam Smith wrote, "As we have no immediate experience of what other men feel, we can form no idea of the manner in which they are affected, but by conceiving what we ourselves should feel in the like situation ... [I]t is by the imagination only that we can form any conception of what are his sensations.... By the imagination we place ourselves in his situation."[19]

Notwithstanding the claim that sympathy was a universal human capacity, most eighteenth-century idealizations implicitly envisioned "humanity" as a masculine figure.[20] Thus if the Enlightenment idea of sympathy was gendered at all, it was gendered as masculine.[21] As the basis for civic virtue and social benevolence, for example, "sympathy" was central to the notion of citizenship, a role described in the distinctly public, masculine terms of "disinterested civic benevolence."[22] Such claims, though cast in the language of universal humanity, in fact located sympathy within the male-gendered public sphere.

But by the late nineteenth century, the political language of sympathy had migrated toward the discursively feminine. In this period discussions of civic virtue were bifurcating along clearly gendered lines: liberal self-interest as a masculine, public virtue, social benevolence and sympathy as its feminine, domesticated, private counterpart. In the dichotomy between self-interest and altruism can be seen "the role of gender in chasing virtue out of the mainstream of liberal thought."[23] Sympathy, sister to virtue, was harried out of the polis and into the household, out of political discourse and into the private, feminine world of friends and family.

The language of sympathy was not only feminized, it was devalued and sentimentalized. Ann Douglas argues, "Sentimentalization . . . was an inevitable part of the self-evasion of a society both committed to laissez-faire industrial expansion and disturbed by its consequences." The relocation of benevolence and sympathy within the feminine sphere at a time when femininity was read as an emblem of political inferiority produced a subtle devaluation of both.[24]

Within the medical profession, too, the meaning assigned to sympathy was gradually reevaluated.[25] In the traditions of Western medical thought, maintaining good health depended both on internal physiological balance and on a resonance between internal physiology and external environment. The metaphor of sympathy supplied a model for both; it also justified the contextual clues sought by the physician as part of any routine diagnostic interview. But by the 1880s, when quantification, experimentalism, and theories of specific etiology began to govern medicine's scientific and professional norms, holistic or nonsomatic scientific models fell out of favor. Bonnie Ellen Blustein describes, for example, the neurologist William Hammond's discomfort with "suggestive therapies" (psychotherapeutics) unless they were grounded in somatic theories of disease. Likewise, neuropathologists throughout the nineteenth century struggled to refine their understanding of the anatomy and physiology of the "sympathetic" nervous system.[26]

In this context, the imprecise language of sympathy lost much of its power. In John Harley Warner's words, physicians "came to think of disorders less as systemic imbalances in the body's natural harmony, and more as complexes of discrete signs and symptoms that could be analyzed, separated and measured in isolation." Indeed physicians were no longer satisfied merely to inquire about and observe the state of their patients' health. Gradually they were trained to seek the precise "data" for concrete explanations of specific disease processes.[27] Sympathy, by virtue of its explanatory vagueness, its inability to define or control the terms of biomedical inquiry, no less than its sentimentality, took on an increasingly problematic status in the emerging scientific culture of medicine.

In nineteenth-century medical dictionaries, changing definitions of sympathy are sensitive indicators of its devaluation. In the medical definition given by Webster's 1828 *American Dictionary of the English Language,* sympathy is defined as "a correspondence of various parts of the body in similar sensations or affections; or an affection of the whole body or some part of it, in consequence of an injury or disease of another part." By 1833, however, when *Dunglison's Medical Dictionary* repeated this definition, it carefully added the phrase "by means unknown." By 1890 John Shaw Billings's authoritative *National Medical Dictionary* defined the word as "a vague term to express the fact that injury or disease of an organ may produce a change in another part which is not directly connected." For the more precisely anatomical modifier, "sympathetic," Billings bestowed a more precise usage: the sympathetic nervous system "consists of small ganglia on either side of [the] spinal column, connected longitudinally with each other (sympathetic nerve), centrally with cerebro-spinal system . . . peripherally sending branches to viscera." *Dunglison's* 1833 entry had simply read, "The epithet sympathetic is given to different nerves."[28]

Lexicography reflected usage. In 1867, for example, in an article on treatment of alcoholism titled "Methomania," Dr. Albert Day reminded his readers that the sufferings of such patients "cannot be endured alone, but must be shared." He counseled, however, against an unhelpful "intrusive sympathy," recommending instead "a generous tolerance mingled with firmness." In the same essay, however, he confidently employed the concept of the "sympathetic reflex" to explain alcoholism as a somatic disease.[29]

The language of sympathy or "fellow-feeling" did continue to inhabit certain domains within late Victorian medical discourse—although it was not unproblematic. Regina Morantz-Sanchez quotes Dr. Henry Hartshorne in 1872 describing the therapeutic relationship as an art of "the quick eye, the receptive ear, and delicate touch, intensified . . . by a warm sympathetic temperament." Hartshorne was speaking to the students of the Woman's Medical College of Pennsylvania and, as Morantz-Sanchez has shown, late Victorian medical culture clearly assigned the art of sympathy to the repertoire of the female practitioner.[30] But Hartshorne's was not the only strand in the skein of professional advice extended to women physicians in the late nine-teenth century. In 1859 Dr. Marie Zakrzewska, soon to become one of America's leading women physicians, addressed the incoming students of the New England Female Medical College in Boston. Describing what she considered the proper motives for the study of medicine, she disdained those women who were:

> impregnated ... with a perpetual sentimentality ... which bears on its banner the inscription of "Sympathy"; sympathy with their fellow mortals of their own sex, with the suffering sisterhood. However absolutely necessary a certain amount of sympathy and compassion may be, to qualify the physician for success in practice, it will never be the right motive from which the student must start. This predominating, sentimentalizing sympathy, will dwarf or confuse the reason ... and will be pernicious to logic.[31]

The differences between these two statements signal a significant disagreement over the professional identity of the physician—male and female—and the relationship between gender and professionalism. They also testify to a shift in the meaning of doctor-patient communication, reflecting what Warner has described as the changing epistemologies of medicine. To reiterate, the discourse of medicine was becoming gendered, and its gender was decidedly masculine. The sentimentalization of "sympathy" was putting it beyond the pale of modern medical professionalism. To be called a "sympathetic" physician was to risk stigmatization as unscientific. This is the context for Zakrzewska's scathing denunciation of sympathy as the prime motive for women's entry into the medical profession and as a blight on the exercise of clinical judgment. For women doctors, in Zakrzewska's view, this was too great a risk.

Despite Zakrzewska's objections, many well-meaning male physicians like Hartshorne—and many female physicians—saw nothing wrong in identifying sympathy with the feminine members of the profession. As Morantz-Sanchez notes, ever since Elizabeth Blackwell first made this equation in the 1840s, the "feminine" art of sympathetic understanding was seen by many as the raison d'être for female physicians. Some, however—Doctors Zakrzewska and Mary Putnam Jacobi, for example—were far-sighted enough to see the danger both to women physicians and to the medical profession of marginalizing the art of interpersonal understanding by gendering it as "feminine." William Osler also understood the difficulty. His 1889 injunction "Aequanimitas" (equanimity) aimed to shield novice practitioners from the depleting effects of sentimentality. Yet as Susan Lederer observes, Osler feared lest the equanimity to "meet the exigencies of practice" be acquired at the cost of "hardening 'the human heart by which we live.' "[32]

By the 1920s, the impact of sympathy's reduced circumstances—like the faded air of Victorian benevolence—could be observed. References to the act of sympathetic understanding still conveyed compassion but, without its ancient roots in physiology, etiology, and therapeutics, it suggested "pity" rather than "generous tolerance."[33] In a 1916 description of the many hospital settings available at Harvard Medical School, the term "sympathy" appears only in a reference to the McLean Hospital's reputation for "kind and sympathetic treatment of the insane," and in a tribute to the "deep sympathies" of Miss Anne Smith Robbins, founder in 1860 of the House of the Good Samaritan for care of the indigent sick.[34] When such well-known physicians as Richard Cabot or Francis Weld Peabody drew on the language of sympathy in the 1920s, they were speaking self-consciously in the accents of an earlier age.[35]

Like Cabot and Ida Cannon, whose development of the field of medical social work occurred during the same period and for many of the same reasons, Peabody worried about the reductive effect of the new professionalism on doctor-patient communication. On the wards of the modern, urban hospital, the patient-as-person and the full meaning of his or her symptoms tended to disappear. In 1926, shortly before his own death from cancer, Peabody delivered an appeal to physicians in training at Harvard. He wrote, "The most common criticism made at present by older practitioners is that young graduates . . . are too 'scientific' and do not know how to take care of patients." To remedy this, Peabody called on the medical profession to revive the art of therapeutic care. This he explicitly framed in the language of "sympathetic understanding":

> Here is a worried, lonely, suffering man, and if you begin by approaching him with sympathy, tact, and consideration, you get his confidence and he becomes your patient. . . . Make time to have little talks with him—and these talks need not always be about his symptoms. Remember that you want to know him as a man, and this means you must know about his family and friend, his work and his play. What kind of person is he—cheerful, depressed, introspective, careless, conscientious, mentally keen or dull? Look out for all the little incidental things you can do for his comfort. These, too, are a part of "the care of the patient."[36]

Peabody here employed the voice of the past. By revitalizing both the moral and diagnostic potential of the doctor-patient relationship, Peabody sought to return it to the center of professional concern. Acknowledging the social etiology of disease, he called for a broader approach to the acquisition of clinical knowledge than the biological reductionism that was beginning to inform the meaning of doctor-patient communication—an approach expressed through the metaphor of sympathy. But by the 1920s the language of sympathy could no longer command the respect needed to accomplish the task Peabody required of it.

Managed Care: Empathy as "Detached Concern"

By the 1920s the language of "sympathetic understanding" had been marginalized both by gendered associations with Victorian sentimentalism and by the triumph of new physiological and etiologic paradigms. The diminished usefulness of "sympathy" within the lexicon of scientific medicine created a linguistic space to which "empathy" could readily be adapted. Nowhere was this more true than in the psychiatric, and especially the psychoanalytic, setting. The latter's potent combination of intimacy and professional authority demanded construction of techniques both to ensure neutrality and to regulate the acquisition of knowledge about patients.

Thus through most of the twentieth century, empathy has been enlisted for the connective work from which "sympathy" had been disqualified, while simultaneously enforcing the *dis*connections, neutrality, and scientific claims essential to psychodynamic psychiatry. Katz's definition accurately portrays the psychiatric perspective: "As a refined scientific technique . . . empathy calls for a pendulum-like action, alternating between subjective involvement and objective detachment."[37] It provided practitioners a means of engaging with the disturbing closeness of their patients while guarding against the distortions of uncontrolled subjectivity.

To some, however, empathy seemed to threaten a giving-way, an unscientific relaxation of the boundaries separating subject from object, a discursively "feminine" and, by definition, unprofessional identification with the "other."[38] That even Freud grappled with this ambiguity is suggested by his early effort to relate empathy to, and distinguish it from, the concept of ego identification. In his 1921 discussion of group psychology, Freud defined identification as "the original form of emotional tie with an object." Empathy, he insisted, "which plays the largest part in our understanding of what is inherently foreign to our ego in other people," should be interpreted as the "intellectual" counterpart to the more "emotional" and "regressive" components of identification.[39]

The first psychoanalytic study addressed exclusively to empathy, "The Psycho-Analytic Method of Observation," was published in 1925 by Theodore Schroeder. As its title suggests, Schroeder placed empathic understanding at the center of psychoanalysis because it represented the closest means of observing, interpreting, and testing observations of the inner world of the patient. In short, it represented a psychoanalytic version of the scientific method. Stanley Jackson has noted that Helene Deutsch in 1926 and Sandor Ferenczi in 1928 both discussed the importance of dislodging from empathy any remnants of the "occult" or the "mystical."[40] But as late as 1953, Otto Fenichel's work *Identification* associated empathy with "feminine" intuition rather than with understanding of a more intellectual sort. Fenichel referred to empathy as "the intuitive grasp of the real psychic states of another person." He asserted that empathy "is closely related to [narcissistic] identification but is not identical with it. [Such] things as a high degree of narcissism or of the passive sexual aim of being loved instead of loving . . . usually accompany this particular gift for intuitive empathy." He concluded, "These considerations make it plausible that in general women are more empathic than men."[41]

Many of the newer generation in psychoanalysis, however, strongly urged a reexamination and wider appreciation of empathy in the therapeutic process. Between 1958 and 1960 three separate papers appeared— by Ralph Greenson, Roy Schafer, and Heinz Kohut—all apparently part of this rehabilitative project. Writing long before the appearance of a fully articulated discourse of gender, gender nevertheless played as important a part in their construal of empathy as it had for Freud and Fenichel. Though differing in their conclusions, all three authors addressed the implications of gender for the legitimacy of empathic knowledge. Greenson began by observing that the concept of empathy was typically ignored or underestimated. Indeed, he suspected "some antagonism between theory and empathy." His analysis of empathic understanding gives some idea of where such ambivalence may have arisen. Greenson proposed, "Empathy begins in [the] non-verbal, skin, touching, intonational relationship of mother and child." He continued, "Empathy and intuition are related. . . . One empathizes to reach feelings; one uses intuition to get ideas. . . . You arrive at the feelings and pictures via empathy, but intuition . . . picks up the clues that empathy gathered." Finally he speculated, "Since empathy originates in the early mother-child nonverbal communications, it has a definite feminine cast. For men to be empathic they must have come to peace with their motherly component."[42]

Schafer, like Freud, was concerned to distance empathy from its feminine associations, principally by emphasizing its cognitive as well as its emotive aspects. "Generative empathy," according to Schafer, "involves comprehending." Comprehension referred to "a process with equally important cognitive and affective aspects." Schafer saw "pity" and "sympathy" as an alliance with what he termed the "passive, feminine, masochistic aspects" of the patient's situation; in contrast, empathy was extolled as a means of reinforcing the patient's "autonomy," a process that "initiates and promotes growth in the subject, the object, and the relationship between them."[43]

In Heinz Kohut, these concerns found even more explicit formulation. Kohut, in the earliest elaboration of empathy in a literature later labeled "self psychology," equated the term with "vicarious introspection" and noted its connection to the fundamental paradox of psychoanalysis: as, in Kohut's words, an "empirical science," psychoanalysis must be capable of making the observations necessary to acquire data, formulate hypotheses, and generate predictions—all within a field of research bounded by the internal, largely obscure workings of the psyche. Necessarily, then, "introspection and empathy are the essential ingredients of psychoanalytic observation."[44] Joan Lang has written that within the field of self psychology empathy is valued because, "it is vital to data-gathering and interpretation; further it is at the center of Kohut's concept of healthy relationships."[45]

Especially in the former sense—as a quasi-empirical methodology—empathy made its deepest contribution to the psychoanalytic literature, both in the work of Kohut and more generally. Common to the works of Greenson, Schafer, and Kohut on empathy had been a desire to enlist empathy into the project of reasserting the empirical, objective, fundamentally *scientific* character of psychoanalysis. Empathy was understood primarily as a technical instrument for observation, a protocol for therapeutic neutrality, and a banner of methodological exclusivity. During the 1940s and 1950s, both Carl Rogers's "client-centered," "nondirective" psychotherapy and Talcott Parsons's studies of the physicians' social role presented, albeit from different directions, strong challenges to psychoanalytic claims to therapeutic uniqueness—Rogers by exporting the term empathy into a quite different practice modality and Parsons by subsuming the psychotherapeutic role under the more general category of "fundamental features of the role of the physician . . . institutionalized long before the days of Freud."[46] Jerome Frank, in a large-scale comparative study of the major schools of psychotherapy, asserted that *all* psychotherapeutics owed their effectiveness as a "healing art" to a set of common characteristics. In his 1973 edition, Frank used the term "empathy" as a synonym for one of these essentials, the expression of nonjudgmental, but warm, understanding of the patient. Judging by Frank's reference to the "widespread misunderstanding" that greeted these conclusions, psychoanalysts may have been spurred into explicit theoretical accounts of "empathic" understanding to counter the challenging and potentially vitiating effect of Parsons's and Frank's generic description of psychoanalytic method.[47]

Thus until the recent integration of feminist, relational, and hermeneutic insights into the psychiatric literature, psychoanalysis was little motivated to reexamine either its claim to a scientific methodology or a conception of empathy adapted to this approach. Within general clinical medicine and medical education, as in psychiatry, the patient-practitioner relationship was increasingly shaped by the conventions of scientific research and professional dominance: the physician as scientist, the patient as object. Described in its most influential form by Parsons in *The Social System* (1951), this relationship relied fundamentally on a model characterized by necessary asymmetry and structured inequality. Parsons saw the sick role as a form of dependency, a disruption, a kind of legitimate deviance. The professional was, therefore, "a technical expert who legitimizes the claim to illness and is responsible for returning the sick person to his normal role in society."[48] Within the Parsonian model the professional would not only sustain but enforce the continued asymmetry of this relationship.

By the early 1960s, however, in a context of concern over the disappearance of the general practitioner, fears of declining access to primary care, an emerging critique of professionalism, and an increased politicization of health care, a definite shift can be detected in medical educators' approach to patient-practitioner relations.[49] In effect, medical educators began to reassert the professional legitimacy of some degree of personal involvement with patients. But in a discourse that equated professionalism with science and science with objectivity, addressing the issue of interpersonal concern created problems of its own. While distancing themselves from Parsonian paternalism, few practitioners were willing to abandon the professional detachment that had long been a source of both professional legitimacy and personal psychic comfort.

Writing in the *Journal of the American Medical Association* on "Sympathy and Empathy" in 1958, the psychiatrist Charles Aring insisted, "One of the most difficult tasks put upon man is reflective (not reflexive) commitment of oneself to another's problem while maintaining his own identity. . . . A subtle and significant feature of a happy medical practice is to remain unencumbered by the patient's problem." The alternative evoked by Aring harkened back to Fenichel: one must vigilantly maintain one's "emotional boundaries." Otherwise, he feared, one risked becoming the sort of "outer-directed" personality described in David Riesman's *The Organization Man*: "taken in by what he has taken in."[50]

To Aring and many others, empathy seemed the ideal mediator between comfort and risk, not only in psychiatry but in all clinical medicine. Perhaps the most widely quoted example can be found in the work of Renée Fox, a student of Talcott Parsons and an influential sociologist of medicine in her own right.[51] In 1963 Fox and psychiatrist Harold Lief published an essay titled "Training for 'Detached Concern' in Medical Students." They began by observing that "it is generally agreed that it is proper to teach the concept of holistic medicine, in which the patient, rather than just his liver, heart, or even his psyche, is the concern of the physician. [This] requires a set of special attitudes and skills, generally termed empathy." The name they gave to their proposed model was "detached concern." Empathy was its linchpin:

> Empathy essentially involves an emotional understanding of the patient, "feeling into" and being on the same "affective wave length" as the patient; at the same time, it connotes an awareness of enough separateness from the patient so that expert medical skills can be rationally applied to the patient's problems. The empathic physician is sufficiently detached or objective in his attitude toward the patient to exercise sound medical judgment and keep his equanimity, yet he also has enough concern for the patient to give him sensitive, understanding care.[52]

The model of "detached concern" thus acknowledged the need for effective and compassionate communication without sacrificing the profession's claims to neutrality and objectivity. Patient and professional remained two "separate" parties. Just as psychiatry tried to address the tension between intimacy and objectivity, medical educators in the 1960s tried to balance the Oslerian ideal of equanimity with an acknowledgment of humane concern for the patient. "Empathy" seemed to provide such a balance, an interactive but fundamentally detached relationship that did not threaten the roles, values, or personal security of a male-gendered professionalism.[53]

Beyond Detached Concern: Empathy as Relational Knowledge

Since the 1970s, feminist and critical social theorists have challenged both the desirability and the possibility of maintaining complete detachment between subject and object, practitioner and patient. The critique of classical epistemology, particularly within hermeneutics and phenomenology, has helped legitimate subjective forms of knowledge such as empathy. Drawing on the work of Charles Taylor, Rabinow and Sullivan describe meaning as *inter*subjective. It "exists for a subject in a situation . . . there are no simple elements of meaning."[54]

Many feminists would agree that knowledge claims are situated, arising from the specific assumptions of the knower. Yet they are uneasy with the relativism sometimes derived from that position—that there is no way to refute knowledge claims. Empathic knowledge is often subject to the same charge. But as Lorraine Code argues, "The fact that perfect, objective knowledge of other people is not possible" hardly demonstrates that no valid knowledge of others can be obtained. Indeed Code claims that knowledge of other persons ought to stand as *the* paradigmatic epistemic model. Uncertainty characterizes knowledge of all sorts; situated knowledge, including empathy, is not only epistemologically valid but is really the best we can do.[55]

The influence of this position has been felt especially in the psychoanalytic literature. Evelyne Schwaber, for example, urges recognition of the therapist-patient "dyadic matrix" as the fundamental "contextual unit" and, like Charles Taylor, calls for abandonment of the strategy of "reality testing" from the perspective of the "external" observer. Rather, she sees the interpretive work of psychotherapy as occurring from within the intersubjective field constituted by the patient and practitioner, relying on "empathy-introspection as the primary mode of data-gathering, suspending the inferential imposition of a reality from without."[56]

George Atwood and Robert Stolorow further extended Schwaber's point, making even more explicit the ambivalent urge of psychoanalysis both to participate in and to transcend the goals and methods of positivist science. They write: "Psychoanalysis is pictured here as a science of the *intersubjective*. . . . The observational stance is always one within, rather than outside, the intersubjective field or 'contextual unit' (Schwaber, 1979) being observed, a fact that guarantees the centrality of introspection and empathy as the methods of observation (Kohut, 1959)."[57] Although they wish to retain the secure imprimatur of empirical science, theirs is a science of uncertainty, approximation, imagination, intuition, ambiguity, and personal risk.

This hermeneutic direction within psychoanalysis may suggest a way out of the artificially gendered dichotomies our culture often imposes on intersubjective practices such as empathy. Many feminists are uneasy about uncritically linking intersubjective epistemologies with biologically "essentialist" claims about the female nature.[58] Traditional Western notions of gender, which associate subjectivity, irrationality, and the emotions with femininity, are no less irksome. Thus when empathy is conceptualized in its popular sense, as primarily affective or intuitive, it is in danger of being essentialized as "feminine," devalued as subjective, and—more troubling—defined as un-"natural" to masculine behavior. When empathy is understood primarily in its cognitive sense, it seems to be reduced to a mere technique of data collection. Without due regard to *both* aspects of empathic knowledge, its potential for genuine responsiveness and reconnection to patients can be lost.

Our task is to reclaim the validity of empathy as intersubjective knowledge without simultaneously marginalizing it. One influential example is the work of Jean Baker Miller, a psychiatrist, founder of Wellesley College's Stone Center for Developmental Services and Studies, and author of the 1976 book *Toward a New Psychology of Women.*[59] Miller is one of the progenitors of the movement within feminist thought to construct an "affiliative" or "relational" psychology by reinterpreting human development in Western culture according to a feminine developmental model. Stressing the affiliative quality of the feminine socialization processes, Miller is careful not to claim that women are more empathic or relational *by nature*. Then, too, she clearly distinguishes these relational qualities from a merging, fusion, or collapse of individual ego boundaries. Indeed one of Miller's priorities, also evident in the work of her Stone Center colleagues, is to counter the assumption that the affiliative qualities that foster empathic skills are signs of ego fragility or psychological dependency. "We all begin life," she writes, "deeply attached to the people around us. Men, or boys, are encouraged to move out of this state. . . . Women are encouraged to remain." But, and this is Miller's central contribution to a discussion of empathic knowing,

> women's great desire for affiliation is both a fundamental strength, essential for social advance and at the same time the inevitable source of many of women's current problems. That is, while women have reached for and already found a psychic basis for a more advanced social existence, they are not able to act fully and directly . . . in a way that would allow it to flourish.

Miller asks, how can women and men "create a way of life that includes serving others without being subservient?"[60]

Miller is mindful of certain dangers: first the potential for harm in unchecked subjectivism—especially in the doctor-patient relationship; second, the still prevalent identification of subjectivity with femininity and our culture's devaluation of both. These dangers have convinced her of the need to define empathy as both a relational and a cognitive process and to insist that it can be cultivated in the individual through a process of social learning. Similarly, she rejects the link between empathy and "loss of identity." Her colleague Judith Jordan explains, "In order to empathize, one must have a well-differentiated sense of self in addition to an appreciation of . . . the sameness of another person. . . . Ego boundary flexibility is important since there is an 'as-if,' trying-out quality to the experience. . . . If either relaxation or restructuring of ego boundaries is impaired, empathy will suffer."[61] What is needed, we are beginning to realize, is a model of empathy in the therapeutic relationship that acknowledges its cognitive, analytic features without sacrificing its attentive qualities.

Within this history of "empathy" one can find the remnants of an older unease with the radical potential of femininity in Western culture. Our cultural bifurcation of "masculine" and "feminine" contributed to the dichotomized meanings assigned to the concept of empathy: a male-gendered, objective, value-neutral technique—a clinical analogue to empirical data collection; or a female-gendered, relational modality. As Miller and Jordan make clear, any reliance on affiliative, empathic, interpersonal knowledge seems to require a disclaimer: adopting this relational modality will not consign one to the margins of professional respectability.

Unfortunately, allowing this contestation of meaning to remain unreconciled threatens to limit the therapeutic usefulness of empathic understanding. If communication between doctor and patient is to overcome the centrifugal forces of gender, race, and social class within modern culture, we will need relational processes like empathy to help restructure our expectations for professional practice.[62] I am convinced that it must be reclaimed for the *human* enterprise of deconstructing the differences and reducing the distances between practitioner and patient in modern health care.

Notes

Many thanks to Martha Holstein, Mary White, and Dr. Katherine Ochsner, graduate students at the Institute for the Medical Humanities, University of Texas Medical Branch; to Professors Theodore Brown, Warren Carrier, Ronald Carson, Tom Cole, Ellen Dwyer, Gerald Grob, Howard Kushner, Maureen Milligan, Susan Reverby, Arleen Tuchman, Harold Vanderpool, and John Harley Warner; and to Drs. Chester Burns, Lucy Candib, Stanley Jackson, Joan Lang, and Richard Selzer for helpful comments on this material.

    1. See the text discussion at note 8.

2. See the text discussion at note 50.

3. Jean Baker Miller, *Toward a New Psychology of Women*, 2nd ed. (1976; Boston: Beacon Press, 1986); Nancy Chodorow, *The Reproduction of Mothering: Psychoanalysis and the Sociology of Women* (Berkeley: University of California Press, 1978); Carol Gilligan, *In a Different Voice: Psychological Theory and Women's Development* (Cambridge, Mass.: Harvard University Press, 1982).

4. See Linda J. Nicholson, ed., *Feminism/Postmodernism* (London: Routledge, 1990). See also Marilyn Hirsch and Evelyn Fox Keller, eds., *Conflicts in Feminism* (New York: Routledge, 1990); Joan Scott, *Gender and the Politics of History* (New York: Columbia University Press, 1988); Martha Minow, *Making All the Difference: Inclusion, Exclusion, and American Law* (Ithaca, N.Y.: Cornell University Press, 1990); Susan Bordo, *The Flight to Objectivity: Essays in Cartesianism and Culture* (Albany: State University of New York Press, 1987); Maureen Milligan, "Reflections on Feminist Scepticism, the 'Maleness' of Philosophy and Postmodernism," *Hypatia* 7:3 (Summer 1992):166–172. See also Evelyn Fox Keller, *Reflections on Gender and Science* (New Haven: Yale University Press, 1985), esp. 99, 107, 117; Paul Rabinow and William M. Sullivan, eds., *Interpretive Social Science: A Second Look* (Berkeley: University of California Press, 1987).

5. James E. Rosenberg and Bernard Towers, "The Practice of Empathy as a Prerequisite for Informed Consent," *Theoretical Medicine* 7 (1986):181–194; Howard M. Spiro, "What Is Empathy and Can It Be Taught?" *Ann. Int. Med.*, 116:10 (1992):843–846. Unfortunately *Empathy and the Practice of Medicine: Beyond Pills and the Scalpel*, ed. Howard M. Spiro, Mary G. McCrea Curnen et al. (New Haven: Yale University Press, 1993) reached me too late for inclusion.

6. Robert L. Katz, *Empathy: Its Nature and Uses* (London: Free Press of Glencoe/Collier-Macmillan, 1963), 1.

7. Lauren G. Wispe, "Sympathy and Empathy," in *International Encyclopedia of the Social Sciences*, ed. David L. Sills (New York: Macmillan, 1968), 441–447. Wispe here adopts the definition of psychologist Carl R. Rogers. Stanley W. Jackson's excellent article, "The Listening Healer in the History of Psychological Healing," *Amer. J. Psych.* 149:12 (December 1992):1623–1632, sets "empathic listening" into the context of nineteenth-century medicine's emphasis on visual observation rather than listening.

8. See, for example, Alfred Margulies, *The Empathic Imagination* (New York: W. W. Norton and Co., 1989).

9. Charles Edward Gauss, "Empathy," in *The Dictionary of the History of Ideas* ed. Philip P. Wiener (New York: Charles Scribner's Sons, 1973), 85–89. For the current German usages, cf. *Langenscheidt Standard Dictionary of the English and German Languages* (1969).

10. Sigmund Freud, *Group Psychology and the Analysis of the Ego*, trans. James Strachey (1921; London: Hogarth Press, 1948), 70n2, also 66. See also the third section below.

11. Gauss, "Empathy," 85–89; Paul Rabinow and William M. Sullivan,

"The Interpretive Turn: A Second Look," in *Interpretive Social Science*, ed. Rabinow and Sullivan, 1–30. For a recent philosophical analysis of empathy, see Lorraine Code, *What Can She Know?* (Ithaca, N.Y.: Cornell University Press, 1991).

12. *The American Heritage Dictionary of the English Language*, 3rd ed. (1992).

13. Gauss, "Empathy," 87.

14. John Harley Warner, *The Therapeutic Perspective: Medical Practice, Knowledge, and Identity in America, 1820–1885* (Cambridge, Mass.: Harvard University Press, 1986). For fine analyses of the current structure of patient-practitioner communication see Sue Fisher, *In the Patient's Best Interest* (New Brunswick, N.J.: Rutgers University Press, 1986); Alexandra Dundas Todd, *Intimate Adversaries: Cultural Conflicts between Doctors and Their Women Patients* (Philadelphia: University of Pennsylvania Press, 1989); Howard Waitzkin, *The Politics of Medical Encounters: How Patients and Doctors Deal with Social Problems* (New Haven: Yale University Press, 1991); and Candace West, *Routine Complications: Troubles with Talk between Doctors and Patients* (Bloomington: Indiana University Press, 1984).

15. Janet Oppenheim, *"Shattered Nerves": Doctors, Patients, and Depression in Victorian England* (New York: Oxford University Press, 1991), 95; Edwin Clarke and L. S. Jacyna, *Nineteenth-Century Origins of Neuroscientific Concepts* (Berkeley: University of California Press, 1987), 102; cf. Owsei Temkin, *The Falling Sickness: A History of Epilepsy from the Greeks to the Beginnings of Modern Neurology*, 2nd ed. rev. (1945; Baltimore: Johns Hopkins University Press, 1971), esp. 60–61, 216, 247–249.

16. John Quincy, M.D., *Lexicon Physico-Medicum; or, A New Medical Dictionary* (London, 1743); Gregory's *Lectures on the Duties and Qualifications of a Physician* (1772) is quoted in Laurence B. McCullough, "Historical Perspectives on the Ethical Dimensions of the Patient-Physician Relationship: The Medical Ethics of Dr. John Gregory," *Ethics in Science and Medicine* 3 (1978):47–53, esp. 49.

17. David Hume, "An Enquiry Concerning the Principles of Morals" (1751; 1777), in *British Moralists, 1650–1800*, vol. 2, ed. D. D. Raphael (1969; Indianapolis: Hackett Publishing Company, 1991), 76; Gordon S. Wood, *The Radicalism of the American Revolution* (New York: Alfred S. Knopf, 1992), 220, 221, 236–240; Annette C. Baier, "Hume: The Woman's Moral Theorist?" in Eva Feder Kittay and Diana T. Meyers, eds., *Women and Moral Theory* (Savage, Md.: Rowman & Littlefield, 1987), 37–55, esp. 41.

18. Annette C. Baier, *A Progress of Sentiments* (Cambridge, Mass.: Harvard University Press, 1991), 50, 53; David Hume, "A Treatise of Human Nature" (1739–40), in *British Moralists*, vol. 2, ed. Raphael, 48–107; Hume, "An Enquiry Concerning the Principles of Morals," ibid., 76; McCullough, "Historical Perspectives," 51.

19. Adam Smith, "The Theory of Moral Sentiments" (1759; 1790), in *British Moralists*, vol. 2, ed. Raphael, 201–202.

20. Laurence McCullough has found that John Gregory's discussion of

"sympathy" is an important exception to these remarks in that Gregory explicitly gendered "sympathy" as feminine. Personal communication, January 27, 1994.

21. See Londa Schiebinger, *The Mind Has No Sex? Women in the Origins of Modern Science* (Cambridge, Mass.: Harvard University Press, 1989), esp. 206–233.

22. Joan C. Williams, "Domesticity as the Dangerous Supplement of Liberalism," *J. Women's History* 2:3 (Winter 1991):69–88; Ruth H. Bloch, "The Gendered Meanings of Virtue in Revolutionary America," *Signs: Journal of Women in Culture and Society*, 13:1 (Autumn 1987):37–58; Joan C. Tronto, *Moral Boundaries: A Political Argument for an Ethics of Care* (New York: Routledge, 1993), esp. chap. 2. Also cf. J.G.A. Pocock, *The Machiavellian Moment: Florentine Political Thought and the Atlantic Republican Tradition* (Princeton: Princeton University Press, 1975).

23. Williams, "Domesticity," 70–77; Wood, *Radicalism*, 218.

24. Ann Douglas, *The Feminization of American Culture* (New York: Alfred A. Knopf, 1978), 12, 48.

25. Lester King, *Transformations in American Medicine* (Baltimore: Johns Hopkins University Press, 1991), 59–61.

26. Clarke and Jacyna, *Nineteenth-Century Origins*, chap. 7 passim, and 102, 320–327, 344–346, 368–369; Bonnie Ellen Blustein, *Preserve Your Love for Science* (New York: Cambridge University Press, 1991), 159–162.

27. Cf. Warner, *The Therapeutic Perspective*, esp. 86–87; Martin S. Pernick, *A Calculus of Suffering: Pain, Professionalism, and Anesthesia in Nineteenth-Century America* (New York: Columbia University Press, 1985).

28. *An American Dictionary of the English Language*, 2 vols., comp. Noah Webster (1828; New York: Johnson Reprint Co., 1970); *Dunglison's Medical Dictionary* (1833); *The National Medical Dictionary*, comp. John S. Billings (Philadelphia: Lea Brothers and Co., 1890). My thanks to Dr. Chester Burns for photocopies of these references from his personal collection.

29. Albert Day, "Methomania," 44, 45, 58, reprinted in Gerald N. Grob, ed., *Nineteenth-Century Medical Attitudes toward Alcoholic Addiction: Six Studies, 1814–1867* (New York: Arno Press, 1981).

30. As quoted in the essay by Regina Morantz-Sanchez in this volume. See also Morantz-Sanchez, *Sympathy and Science: Women Physicians in American Medicine* (New York: Oxford University Press, 1985), esp. chap. 7.

31. Quoted in Arleen Tuchman, in "Gender and Scientific Medicine at a Crossroad? Marie Elizabeth Zakzrewska and the Culture of Medicine," paper presented at the meeting of the American Association for the History of Medicine, Seattle, May 3, 1992.

32. As quoted by Susan E. Lederer in this volume.

33. Day, "Methomania," 50.

34. *The Harvard Medical School and Its Clinical Opportunities*, comp. and ed. Leroy E. Parkins (Boston: Ralph W. Hadley, 1916), 34, 43.

35. Richard C. Cabot, "James Gregory Mumford, M.D.," *Boston Med. Surg.*

J. 172:13 (1915):470–473, esp. 472; Thomas Franklin Williams, "Cabot, Peabody, and the Care of the Patient," *Bull. Hist. Med.* 24 (1950):462–481.

36. Francis Weld Peabody, "Lecture to Medical Students about Patient Care," JAMA 88 (March 19, 1927):877–882. T. Franklin Williams, "Cabot, Peabody, and the Care of the Patient," *Bull. Hist. Med.* 24 (1950):462–481. In this discussion I have profited from reading a section of a forthcoming book by Dr. Lucy Candib.

37. Katz, *Empathy,* 27.

38. The phenomenologist Max Scheler, in *The Nature of Sympathy* (1913), had distinguished between "true" sympathy and the more pathological "identification" which, he believed, was found among "primitive peoples, children, dreamers, neurotics of a certain type, hypnotic subjects and in the exercise of the maternal instinct." See Katz, *Empathy,* 60–63.

39. Sigmund Freud, *Group Psychology and the Analysis of the Ego,* trans. James Strachey (1921; London: Hogarth Press, 1948), 60–71, esp. 65, 66, 70n2.

40. Jackson, "The Listening Healer," 1626–1627, 1631 ref. 27.

41. As quoted in R. Schafer, "Generative Empathy in the Treatment Situation," *Psycho. Qtly.* 28:3 (1959):342–373.

42. R. Greenson, "Empathy and Its Vicissitudes," *Intl. J. Psycho.* 41 (1960): 418–424, esp. 423; Leston Havens, *Making Contact: Uses of Language in Psychotherapy* (Cambridge, Mass.: Harvard University Press, 1986), 16–17.

43. Schafer, "Generative Empathy," 344–346, 364.

44. Heinz Kohut, "Introspection, Empathy, and Psychoanalysis," *J. Amer. Psycho. Assoc.* 7 (1959):459–483. This paper was originally presented in 1957.

45. Joan A. Lang, "Self Psychology and the Understanding and Treatment of Women," *Rev. of Psych.* 9 (1989):390–408, esp. 401. Also see Morton Shane and Estelle Shane, "Self Psychology after Kohut: One Theory or Many?" *J. Amer. Psycho. Assoc.* 41:3 (1993):777–797.

46. Talcott Parsons, "Illness and the Role of the Physician: A Sociological Perspective," *Amer. J. Orthopsych.* 21:1 (1951):452–460, esp. 458–459. Theodore Brown's suggestion that empathy's history was partially shaped by intra-professional tensions within psychiatry merits further study.

47. Jerome D. Frank, *Persuasion and Healing: A Comparative Study of Psychiatry,* rev. ed. (1961; Baltimore: Johns Hopkins University Press, 1973), xvi, 128–130, 214, 324–328. The index of Frank's 1961 edition did not include an entry for "empathy." Cf. 72–73, 192–197. I owe the reference to Frank to Professor Gerald Grob.

48. Samuel W. Bloom and Pamela Summey, "Models of the Doctor-Patient Relationship: A History of the Social System Concept," in *The Doctor-Patient Relationship in the Changing Health Scene,* ed. Eugene B. Gallagher (Washington, D.C.: Department of Health, Education, and Welfare, 1978), 17–41.

49. See Eliot Freidson, *Profession of Medicine* (Chicago: University of Chicago Press, 1970). Also cf. David J. Rothman, *Strangers at the Bedside* (New York: Basic Books, 1991), chap. 6.

50. Charles D. Aring, "Sympathy and Empathy," *JAMA* 167:4 (1958): 448–452. Lief and Fox's discussion of "detached concern," discussed below, relied in part on Aring.

51. For Fox's connection to the work of Talcott Parsons, see Frederic W. Hafferty, *Into the Valley: Death and the Socialization of Medicial Students* (New Haven: Yale University Press, 1991), 14, 15.

52. Harold I. Lief and Renee C. Fox, "Training for 'Detached Concern' in Medical Students," in *The Psychological Basis of Medical Practice*, ed. Harold I. Lief (New York: Harper and Row, 1963), 12–35. Also see M. Daniels, "Affect and Its Control in the Medical Intern," *Amer. J. Soc.* 66 (1960):259–267.

53. Hafferty, *Into the Valley*, 14, 15.

54. Paul Rabinow and William M. Sullivan, "The Interpretive Turn: A Second Look," in *Interpretive Social Science*, ed. Rabinow and Sullivan, 1–30, esp. 7; Charles Taylor, "Interpretation and the Sciences of Man" (1971), reprinted in *Interpretive Social Science*, ed. Rabinow and Sullivan, 33–81.

55. Code, *What Can She Know?*, 82; Camilla Stivers, "Reflections on the Role of Personal Narrative in Social Science," *Signs* 18:2 (1993):408–425, esp. 410.

56. Evelyne Schwaber, "Empathy: A Mode of Analytic Listening," *Psycho. Inquiry* 1:3 (1981):357–392.

57. George E. Atwood and Robert D. Stolorow, *Structures of Subjectivity: Explorations in Psychoanalytic Phenomenology* (Hillsdale, N.J.: Analytic Press, 1984), 41. See also Margulies, *The Empathic Imagination*.

58. Marianne Hirsch and Evelyn Fox Keller, ed., *Conflicts in Feminism* (New York and London: Routledge, 1990); Candace West, "Reconceptualizing Gender in Physician-Patient Relationships," *Soc. Sci. Med.* 36:1 (1993):57–66.

59. Jean Baker Miller, *Toward a New Psychology of Women*, 2nd ed. (1976; Boston: Beacon Press, 1986).

60. Miller, *Toward a New Psychology of Women*, 86, 72.

61. Judith V. Jordan, Janet L. Surrey, and Alexandra G. Kaplan, "Women and Empathy: Implications for Psychological Development and Psychotherapy," in *Women's Growth in Connection: Writings from the Stone Center* (Boston: Guilford Press, 1991), 27–50, esp. 27, 29, 37.

62. See Howard B. Beckman and Richard M. Frankel, "The Effect of Physician Behavior on the Collection of Data," *Annals of Internal Medicine* 101 (1984):692–696; Anthony L. Suchman and Dale A. Matthews, "What Makes the Doctor-Patient Relationship Therapeutic? Exploring the Connexional Dimension of Medical Care," *Ann. Int. Med.* 108 (1988):125–130.

REGINA MORANTZ-SANCHEZ

The Gendering of Empathic Expertise
How Women Physicians Became More Empathic than Men

For more than a decade feminist scholars have critically examined our culture's commonplace notion that women are more empathic than men. They have noted that caring labor is performed primarily by women, and have asked why that has been so.[1] What can the historian offer to these deliberations? In particular, do we find anything in the historical record that can tell us about the development of a concept of empathic expertise in medicine? In answering this question in the affirmative, I intend to highlight aspects of the careers of two very different women physicians who achieved public distinction at the end of the nineteenth century. One, Elizabeth Blackwell, was a founder of the woman's medical movement in the United States and in England, and spent much of her life formulating and disseminating her ideas regarding women physicians' role in society. The other, Mary Dixon-Jones, was a pioneer gynecological surgeon who practiced in Brooklyn, and is the only woman I am aware of who gained entrée to the small, transnational group of elite physicians attempting to shape the direction of gynecology.

The two women did not know each other. Had they met, I doubt whether they could have spent more than five minutes in the same room without coming to verbal blows. Whereas Blackwell thought deeply about the implications of the changes in medicine that were occurring because of the bacteriological revolution, worrying not just about women's role but about the future of patient care more generally, Dixon-Jones embraced those changes with single-minded enthusiasm; her raison d'être was to see to it that she was an integral part of them.

By locating my subjects within their particular social spaces and networks of communication, I will say something about the fate of what we now call "empathy" in the changing medical world of the nineteenth century. In addition, I hope to explore the ways in which representations of gender constituted an important element in the discourse of each of the professional communities of which these two women were a part, thereby coloring conceptions of professionalism and the obligations of physicians to patients.

Elizabeth Blackwell completed her medical training at mid-century, when the role of the physician was shaped by a traditional system of belief and behavior that still explained sickness not as the specific affliction of a particular part of the body but as a condition affecting the entire organism. Therapy was consequently designed to treat the whole patient; the science of medicine lay with the doctor's ability to select the proper drug in the proper dose to bring about the proper physiological effect. To be sure, this task required a thorough knowledge of the therapeutic armamentarium, but it demanded "art" as well: the good practitioner was familiar with the patient's unique personal history and familial influences, all of which were assessed. Physicians treated patients in their own homes, a social context that emphasized the sacredness of personal ties with clients and the relevance of family history to clinical judgments.[2]

Though this system was labeled "scientific," Blackwell and her contemporaries understood the word "science" differently than we do today. For example, few physicians in the nineteenth century would have ignored the importance of intuitive or subjective factors in successful diagnosis and treatment. "The model of the body, health and disease," Charles Rosenberg has written, "was all inclusive, antireductionist, capable of incorporating every aspect of man's life in explaining his physical condition. Just as man's body interacted continuously with his environment, so did his mind with his body, his morals with his health. The realm of causation in medicine was not distinguishable from the realm of meaning in society generally."[3] Blackwell's colleague at the Woman's Medical College of Pennsylvania, Professor Henry Hartshorne, who held a professorship of hygiene similar to the one Blackwell had created for herself at the Woman's Medical College of the New York Infirmary, could have been speaking for her when he observed in an 1872 commencement address, "It is not always the most logical, but often the most discerning physician who succeeds best at the bedside. Medicine is indeed, a science, but its practice is an art. Those who bring the quick eye, the receptive ear, and delicate touch, intensified, all of them, by a warm sympathetic temperament . . . may use the learning of laborious accumulators, often, better than they themselves could do."[4]

Blackwell's professional community consisted primarily of physicians and social reformers who held there to be a social, political, and moral component to sickness. The good physician addressed not only the health of the body but the health of the body politic. When advances in Parisian physiology during the first third of the century discredited much of traditional therapeutics, revealing the self-limiting quality of much disease, some practitioners, Blackwell included, responded by emphasizing the importance of preventive medicine. Many saw hygienic management as the best means of furthering clinical medicine, and some applied this logic by advocating public prevention as a way out of the excessive skepticism and therapeutic gloom of mid-nineteenth-century medical practice. Henry Bowditch of Harvard Medical School, for example, believed that the physician of the future would be concerned primarily with education, on both the individual and the state level.[5]

For others, the dramatic bacteriological discoveries in the last decades of the nineteenth century led to a new paradigm of experimental science. Not only had researchers isolated pathogenic bacteria for numerous epidemic diseases, but they offered a new ideology of science in medicine consisting of an acceptance of the germ theory, the isolation and identification of specific diseases, increasing specialization within medical practice, and a growing willingness to resort to evidence produced in the laboratory. While older practitioners continued to emphasize the importance of clinical observation and the inevitability of individual differences in treatment, laboratory enthusiasts argued that the chemical and physiological principles derived from experimentation must inform therapeutics. Patient idiosyncrasies and environmental differences were gradually stripped of their significance, while reductionist and universalistic criteria for treatment took their place. The experimental therapeutist focused less on the patient and more on the physiological process under investigation. The result was a competing definition of what constituted science in medicine and "a thoroughgoing rearrangement of the relationships among therapeutic practice, knowledge, and professional identity."[6]

Elizabeth Blackwell did not share the high hopes accompanying the new discoveries in the laboratory and remained suspicious of their usefulness. Others in her professional community also rejected the new medical materialism, clinging to traditional antireductionist approaches to patient care. Several historians, indeed, have demonstrated how and in what ways laboratory medicine threatened more traditional epistemological categories.[7] But what is especially intriguing about Blackwell's critique is that her arguments drew on the language of domesticity. Moreover, her thinking about medicine was deeply influenced by her conceptions of gender. Her writings about the good practitioner framed a discourse about gender that privileged empathic expertise over the new science of the laboratory and associated the one with women and the other with men.

At the core of the nineteenth-century ideology of domesticity was the concept of the moral mother. The female qualities of nurturing, sympathy, and moral superiority were depicted as naturally flowing from the experience of maternity. As the family was romanticized, women were increasingly depicted at its moral and spiritual center and assigned a pivotal place in the preservation of values intended to inform not only family life but the social institutions of society at large. In addition, women's elevated moral status was integrally connected to their disinterestedness. "Only by giving up all self-interest and 'living for others,'" Joan Williams has observed, "could women achieve the purity that allowed them to establish moral reference points for their families and for society at large."[8]

Elizabeth Blackwell believed that motherhood, much like the practice of medicine itself, was a "remarkable specialty" because of the "spiritual principles" that underlay the ordinary tasks most mothers performed daily. These she called "the spiritual power of maternity," and they informed both her notions of moral responsibility and her formulations of what constituted good science. Indeed, for Blackwell this power had much in common with the psychologist Erik Erikson's idea of generativity, a concern for ensuring the healthy moral and physical growth of the next generation. Not only physicians but all mankind must learn to harness it. Moreover, the insights that could be derived from the social practice of mothering could not be measured or reproduced in the laboratory.[9]

The microbe hunters posed three fundamental dangers to medicine as Blackwell understood it. First, their conception of disease etiology was reductionistic and materialistic. Although medicine deserved to be called scientific, the definition of science must not be forced within the narrow confines of bacteriology's deterministic model. Science is not, she insisted, "an accumulation of isolated facts, or of facts torn from their natural relations. . . . Science . . . demands the exercise of our various faculties as well as of our senses. . . . Scientific method requires that all the factors which concern the subject of research shall be duly considered. . . . [For example] the facts of affection, companionship, sympathy, justice . . . exercise a powerful influence over the physical organization of all living creatures."[10]

Blackwell's second objection was to the practice of vivisection, an experimental tool essential to laboratory physiology. It was not so much the plight of animals that concerned her but the process of detachment from the object of research that experiments on live animals inevitably encouraged. She believed such laboratory experiences would harden medical students and inure them to "that intelligent sympathy with suffering, which is a fundamental quality in the good physician." Soon, she predicted, they would be regarding the sick poor simply as "clinical material." In addition, Blackwell believed that laboratory research stimulated the increase in gynecological surgery, which rendered more and more women incapable of having children.[11]

These two fundamental objections inevitably led Blackwell to her third: the fear that a preoccupation with the laboratory would turn the profession away from an emphasis on clinical practice and severely threaten the doctor-patient relationship. Although research was indispensable to the physician's task, it must be focused on the patient, not on abstract physiological laws, and certainly not on the physiology of animals. Like other colleagues similarly contending with changes in medicine, Blackwell emphasized behavior over biomedical knowledge as the basis for professional identity. More important than long hours in the laboratory were a physician's skills in clinical observation and the ability to maintain "character" at the bedside. "It is not a brilliant theorizer that the sick person requires," she reminded her students, "but the experience gained by careful observation and sound commonsense, united to the kindly feeling and cheerfulness which make the very sight of the doctor a cordial to the sick." The "true" physician had two obligations to the patient: to cure disease and to relieve suffering through empathy, or what she and most Victorians called "sympathy."[12]

We need not invoke the etymology of the word "empathy" or consult its complex contemporary definitions to understand that Blackwell's notion of empathic expertise was essential to her concept of professionalism. By modeling the doctor-patient relationship on the interaction between mother and child, Blackwell was clearly gendering such behavior, though she was careful to assert that it was something that men could learn. She went even further in her elaboration of gender dualisms, however, when she labeled the new science "male." Indeed, she blamed bacteriology on the "male intellect," and warned her students against the tyranny of male authority in medicine. "It is not blind imitation of men, nor thoughtless acceptance of whatever may be taught by them that is required," she wrote. Women students, she regretted, were as yet too "accustomed to accept the government and instruction of men as final, and it hardly occurs to them to question it." They must be taught that "methods and conclusions formed by one-half the race only, must necessarily require revision as the other half of humanity rises into conscious responsibility."[13]

Blackwell's critique of bacteriology through the invocation of culturally available gender symbols represented a contestation of changing power relationships in medicine. The association of empathic behavior with femininity was something relatively new.[14] When we recall the comments of Henry Hartshorne cited at the beginning of this essay, we are reminded of an older concept of professional behavior that maintained a place for intuition and sympathy and stressed the therapeutic powers of moral and social concerns. Drawing on aspects of this older tradition, Blackwell also seems to have been reformulating it by valorizing a certain kind of clinical behavior and connecting it with women. What is implicit but not stated is that objectivity and professional disengagement—qualities intensely identified with the new version of scientific medicine—are male. Ironically, though her intention was to mount a critique of the changes in medicine, defining a particular form of behavior as female may have had exactly the opposite of her intended effect, because it linked interpersonal concern with a subordinate social group.[15]

Indeed, it seems that Blackwell was losing her audience. Her faultfinding with the new ideology of science reached a relatively small and circumscribed group of male and female practitioners, most of whom were losing ground in the face of rapid changes in the organization and practice of medical care. Although women physicians welcomed her ideas about the unique qualities they had to offer the profession, in part because the argument proved a still powerful justification for their occupational aspirations, more and more of them found her critique of the new science irrelevant to their experience.

It would be difficult to find a woman physician for whom Blackwell's discourse on medicine had less resonance than Mary Dixon-Jones. A graduate of the Woman's Medical College of Pennsylvania in 1873 at the age of forty-five, and only seven years younger than Blackwell, Jones's circuitous path to her profession was a familiar one for women physicians of that first generation. She began as a teacher, taught physiology at various female seminaries, and read medicine with a well-known Maryland physician, Dr. Thomas Bond. In the 1860s she received a sectarian medical degree from a hydropathic college in New York.

But like several women physicians in those early years who attended sectarian institutions because no regular medical school would accept them, Jones found herself drawn back into medical study later in her career, this time at an orthodox institution. She spent three years in the early 1870s matriculating in Philadelphia at the Woman's Medical College, displaying a particular interest in microscopy and pathology. In 1873 she passed a three-month preceptorship in New York with Mary Putnam Jacobi, a highly respected and Paris-trained woman physician and medical professor, and later took courses at the New York Postgraduate Medical School.

It was probably during this period that Dixon-Jones came into contact with the new science of bacteriology. Moreover, as a student at the Woman's Medical College, she no doubt attended surgical clinics at Blockley Hospital and studied surgery with Professor Emmeline Horton Cleveland, another Paris-trained woman physician who was also dean of the school for two of the three years that Jones was there. A highly skilled technician and beloved by her students, Cleveland was the first woman surgeon to perform an ovariotomy in Philadelphia.[16]

One of the earliest by-products of the new experimental science occurred primarily in the operating room. While the gradual use of anesthesia after mid-century had lessened the pain of surgery, Lister's adaptation of the germ theory in developing the principles of antisepsis had guaranteed the relatively safe surgical invasion of the body for a variety of hitherto incurable complaints. Many of these were gynecological; by far the largest proportion of abdominal operations between 1860 and the end of the 1890s were performed on women.

Jones must have watched these developments keenly, because in 1881 she became the chief medical officer of the Women's Dispensary and Hospital of the city of Brooklyn, a charitable organization whose Board of Lady Managers boasted some of the most prominent matrons in the city. Heightening discord with the hospital's board, however, probably over her increasing interest in ovariotomy, led to a severing of that professional relationship in January 1884. A few months later she established her own gynecological hospital, an institution that allowed her complete autonomy and flexibility in the medical decision-making process, since she dominated its Board of Trustees.

In the beginning the hospital was called the J. Marion Sims Hospital and Dispensary, though its name was soon changed to the Woman's Hospital of Brooklyn. The original name is revealing of Dixon-Jones's apparent desire to identify herself with the recently deceased pioneer gynecological surgeon of New York City, who had successfully presided over a revolution in gynecological surgery with the founding of the New York Woman's Hospital in the 1850s.[17] Much like many other would-be specialists in surgical gynecology, both in the United States and England, Dixon-Jones's relationship with a specialty hospital—in her case, the Woman's Hospital of Brooklyn—was crucial to her professional career. The rise of specialty hospitals like hers in Brooklyn was an important chapter in the development of gynecology in this period.[18]

Specialty hospitals provided a means for particularly ambitious practitioners to make a mark in their chosen field. Although the profession as a whole was skeptical of specialization, proponents justified their work by hailing the process of division of labor in medicine. By the end of the century, at least where women's hospitals were concerned, most practitioners had conceded the point of Dr. Charles Routh, a founding member of the British Gynaecological Society, who emphasized how important specialty hospitals were to the study of specific diseases. "Instead of three, four . . . there were . . . a hundred, or two hundred patients. The medical attendant could, therefore, reason on all of them. . . . No man could come to any positive conclusion as to the treatment of special diseases till he had many examples."[19]

As a woman, of course, Dixon-Jones's interest in surgery could not have been pursued with much success at any of the existing hospitals, except those few connected with a woman's medical school. For example, though the Board of Lady Managers at J. Marion Sims's New York Hospital had stipulated that he appoint a woman assistant, Sims neglected to do so, and it was well into the twentieth century before a woman surgeon operated at the hospital he founded.

Jones's hospital was small, with perhaps only ten to fifteen beds, and seems to have been devoted almost exclusively to gynecological surgery. The medical staff consisted of Jones, her son Charles, a recent graduate of the New York College of Physicians and Surgeons, and another woman physician from the Woman's Medical College of Pennsylvania, Dr. Eliza J. Chapin-Minard. Both her son and Minard assisted Jones in her operations.

Once she had established her own hospital, Dixon-Jones both pursued her specialty and went about the task of meticulously constructing a professional identity in gynecological surgery and surgical pathology. Indeed, she was an aggressive self-promoter who instinctively moved to counteract the obvious barriers to advancement that presented themselves to an aspiring female surgeon. In the spring of 1884 she performed her first laparotomy, removing a diseased ovary and its appendages from a woman she diagnosed as a classic case of "hystero-epilepsy due to reflex irritation."[20] Four cases of ovariotomy followed the next year, and seven the year after that. In 1886 she made an extended visit to Europe, studying and making herself known in various hospitals and visiting the clinics of some of the most reknowned surgeons, including Lawson Tait, Theodore Bilroth, August Martin,

Carl Schroeder, and Jules Péan. Upon her return the following year, she performed thirty-six ovariotomies and is credited with completing the first total hysterectomy for fibroid tumor ever attempted in the United States.[21]

Along with her surgical accomplishments, Dixon-Jones continued her interest in pathology, carefully studying microscopically tumors and tissue removed from the bodies of her patients. She developed an intimate acquaintance with Dr. Carl Heitzman, a Hungarian immigrant who was known as an expert microscopist and was a specialist in skin diseases.[22] He aided her in making slides and preparing specimens, and she accomplished much of her scientific work under his guidance. She became a member of the New York Pathological Society and frequently brought in specimens for discussion. Beginning in 1884, she commenced publishing pathological findings and clinical case reports in leading journals such as the *American Journal of Obstetrics,* the *Medical Record,* and the *British Gynaecological Journal,* thereby calling attention to herself both as a technical virtuoso in the operating room and as a careful scientist in the laboratory. During her lifetime she published more than thirty papers in gynecology and surgery. Indeed, the *Dictionary of American Medical Biography* credits her not only with being the first U.S. surgeon to perform a total hysterectomy for uterine myoma but also with describing and identifying two diseases—endothelioma, cancer of the lining of the uterus, and gyroma, a cancerous tumor of the ovary.[23]

Dixon-Jones successfully used her medical articles to create the sense among her readers that she was a member of a relatively small group of elite gynecological practitioners in the United States and Europe who were pioneering in operative approaches to women's diseases. Her first article, for example, entitled "A Case of Tait's Operation," was a rather audacious attempt to associate her work with the world-renowned ovariotomist from Birmingham, England, Lawson Tait. She continued to reference Tait over and over again in subsequent publications. She corresponded with him as well, printing part of one of his letters to her in a footnote to one article and telling her readers in another that her son Charles had served as his "first assistant" in 1886, when they made a grand European tour. She eventually attracted Tait's attention sufficiently to prompt him to refer to her at length in one of his own publications.[24]

But it was not only Tait with whom she persistently identified in her published work. Her articles mention connections, conversations, and consultations with elite gynecological surgeons in New York, Boston, and Philadelphia, and demonstrate familiarity with the work of most of the well-known ovariotomists who published in the leading journals. Her articles were characterized by incessant name dropping, coupled with continuous self-referencing to other of her publications and frequent claims to being "the first" to discover a particular cell formation or to try a certain procedure. In terms of her self-presentation, Dixon-Jones was a person who had succeeded in the world of gynecological surgery, someone who embraced and understood the new science.

Ironically, the aggressiveness with which she orchestrated her own success probably hastened her downfall. In April 1889, Dixon-Jones sent a note to the Brooklyn *Eagle* requesting that the paper print a feature story on her hospital in order to "draw public attention to its good works." The institution, she explained, drew its clientele primarily from the urban poor and depended on a combination of city charity funds and private donations. Mysteriously, that very day the newspaper received an anonymous communication accusing Jones of running a private enterprise with public funds. With the certainty of Greek tragedy, Dixon-Jones's plan to promote herself and her hospital soon began to backfire.

A reporter assigned to investigate eventually crafted a series of unflattering articles about Dixon-Jones that touched off an avalanche of public criticism and resulted in two manslaughter charges and eight malpractice suits against her. The articles implied that she was an ambitious and self-promoting social climber, a knife-happy, irresponsible surgeon who forced unnecessary operations on innocent and unsuspecting women and used the specimens gleaned from them to advance her reputation in diagnosis and pathology. Although the first manslaughter case ended in acquittal and the rest of the charges were eventually dropped, the court battles took four years. In 1892 Dixon-Jones attempted to restore her reputation by charging the *Eagle* with libel.

Her lawyers sought $300,000 in damages, claiming that their client had been victimized by the newspaper, aided by certain disreputable members of Brooklyn's medical establishment. A legal spectacle of major proportions, the ensuing trial involved some of the most prestigious physicians in New York and Brooklyn. Medical journals and leading newspapers covered it daily. Testimony took almost two months; roughly three hundred witnesses were called, including former patients with babies in their arms. Jars full of specimens and surgical mannequins became common sights in the courtroom. When Jones lost the case, the state and city withdrew public funds from her hospital and its charter was revoked. Being deprived of her operating theater effectively ended Mary Dixon-Jones's surgical career. Relocating to New

York City, she became an editor of the *Woman's Medical Journal* and passed the decade and a half before her death publishing articles on pathology, utilizing over and over again the specimens and slides collected from the hundred or so operations she had performed in the previous decade.

The trial testimony is a gold mine of complex and interrelated themes. We learn much about Dixon-Jones's status within the Brooklyn medical community, her relationship with a self-created group of elite gynecological surgeons in New York City and elsewhere, and the tensions over specialization seething within the profession at large. I concentrate here, however, on the ways in which representations of gender became embedded in the construction of new professional identities.

In retrospect, it is clear that Dixon-Jones's behavior offended professional colleagues in Brooklyn from the very beginning. In the spring of 1884, for example, her application for membership in the King's County Medical Society was tabled on the grounds that "there is so much opposition to her name that it would be well to postpone action."[25] In contrast, her son Charles did become a member in good standing and remained so until 1892, despite his role as her surgical assistant. Dr. Landon Carter Gray testified that he had initially advocated Dixon-Jones's admission into the society. But he had been told by several colleagues that she had a poor reputation, though he "knew [of] no instance of unprofessional conduct on her part." Others who took the stand to respond to questions regarding her professional standing were equally vague.[26]

To complicate matters further, Dixon-Jones's medical detractors were not all male. Several women physicians, at least two of whom were members of the county medical society, voiced reservations regarding her medical reputation. Caroline S. Pease, an 1877 graduate of the Woman's Medical College of Pennsylvania, claimed that she had worked as Dixon-Jones's assistant briefly in 1886, and detected in her practice "a very marked discrimination" in favor of surgical cases.

Eliza Mosher and her partner Lucy Hall Brown also took the witness stand to express reservations about Dixon-Jones's character. In a letter to her friend and mentor Elizabeth Blackwell, written the week Dixon-Jones's first case report appeared in the *American Journal of Obstetrics*, Mosher reported, no doubt referring to Jones: "There are several regularly graduated women who are already members of the Kings Co. Med. Soc. There is one who, judging from her paper read before the Pathological Soc. not long since, is rather an able woman, but her manners are beyond description—we could not identify our selves with her safely and she is an element of evil because of her coarseness."[27]

One can only surmise what behavioral traits Mosher was referring to, but several witnesses and the newspaper itself drew a portrait of a strong-willed and outspoken woman who was not above tongue-lashing uncooperative colleagues and laypersons. A.J.C. Skene, for example, confessed that Dixon-Jones threatened him when he ceased consulting with her, warning him that "she had a tongue and would use it."[28] Even Kelly and Burrage, the authors of the *Dictionary of American Medical Biography*, published long after her death, remarked on Dixon-Jones's reputation for giving offense. They noted that Jones was "peculiar in person," "flashy and tawdry in appearance," and speculated that "lack of judgment and of intimate contact with the better members of the profession may have been responsible for a certain mental obliquity with which she is accredited."[29]

Expert medical testimony at the trial suggests that at least some of this professional hostility came from conservative Brooklyn physicians who not only disapproved of Jones's celebration of surgical solutions to pelvic disease but remained suspicious of the direction gynecology had moved in the last two decades. At the heart of the matter was tension over specialization, which continued to gain momentum in the second half of the nineteenth century. Suspicion of specialists in medicine had deep historical roots, given that specialization before this period had always been associated with quackery. But in the last decades of the century it became associated with the new ideology of science, which tended to deemphasize holistic approaches to disease in favor of localized pathological anatomy.

The work of the Paris school in the 1830s and 1840s, for example, proved crucial to the development of gynecological surgery, because researchers increasingly tended to break down the body into its component parts. New technology such as the stethoscope and the thermometer and new techniques such as auscultation, percussion, and palpation allowed practitioners to concentrate on specific organs or abnormal internal structures and develop new approaches to treatment. Ovariotomies could not have been attempted, Jane Sewall reminds us, "without a clear concept of local pathological anatomy—without believing that a woman with a grossly distended abdomen had ovarian lesions."[30]

When anesthesia and antisepsis greatly increased the safety of surgery in the 1860s, the traditional criteria for operations—that surgery should be resorted to only in life-threatening situations—seemed no longer justifiable. Gynecological surgeons were among that segment of the physician population who became impatient with palliative treatment—primarily draining and tapping—which rarely offered permanent solutions to patients whose lives were blighted by chronic disease.

The men who created the specialty of surgical gynecology tended to be young and ambitious. They were bucking medical tradition in a number of ways, and their interest in women's diseases was stimulated substantially by the fact that surgical gynecology afforded them a place in the profession. Perhaps it is also worth pointing out that the gradual shift from art to science, from general practice to specialization, echoes in a very real sense the anxieties generated by the transition from craft traditions, where unique products were fashioned holistically by a skilled workman, to mass production, where uniform products were produced in a reductionist manner by a series of "specialists" created by the division of labor. Dixon-Jones's self-promotion, her making of herself into a professional commodity, is part of such a transformation.[31]

The successful ascendancy of surgical treatment led to a decided power shift in the medical hierarchy. The ambitious and entrepreneurial approach to professional disputes displayed by gynecological surgeons prompted more traditional physicians to lament the passing of an older, gentlemanly image. Suspicion of the new professional style can be detected in the outcry against specialization as elitist and dehumanizing; indeed, similar accusations were hurled against laboratory science, and it is no coincidence that Elizabeth Blackwell spoke disparagingly of both in the same breath.

One hears echoes of these controversies in the Dixon-Jones trial testimony. Dixon-Jones's critics, all of whom practiced in Brooklyn, focused primarily on the uncertain validity of her therapeutics and on her questionable professional "character." The testimony of A.J.C. Skene was typical. Known to be a staunch conservative on the subject of ovariotomy, Skene was professor of gynecology at the Long Island College Hospital and a recognized authority on women's diseases. He acknowledged that he had known Dixon-Jones for fifteen or sixteen years, that she had operated on two of his patients against his recommendation, and that he no longer consulted with her. When Jones's lawyer tried to characterize Skene as a member of the "conservative" as opposed to the "radical" school of gynecology, Skene demurred, commenting that with good surgeons "surgery was never resorted to except in cases where life would be in danger if no operation should be performed."[32] Others questioned Dixon-Jones's pathological diagnoses, implying that she had invented them after the fact merely to justify her resort to the knife.[33]

In defense of Jones came an array of prominent surgeons from New York City and Philadelphia. A. M. Phelps, W. Gill Wylie, and H. Marion Sims each confirmed that they had done hundreds of laparotomies of the type performed by Jones, and that they had consulted with her on numerous occasions. Wylie observed that the danger of laparotomy "had now become so slight that much less ceremony was observed than there used to be."[34]

What is particularly striking about this testimony is its subtext. One does not get the feeling from these statements that the speakers were particularly close to Dixon-Jones or had an interest in promoting her. Yet these prominent practitioners, some of them at the pinnacle of their careers, traveled across the Brooklyn Bridge at considerable personal inconvenience to give evidence on behalf of a woman. In theory, they were no more accepting of women physicians than any other of their male colleagues.[35] But they quickly grasped that it was not simply Dixon-Jones's surgical career that was on trial but theirs as well. In this instance, gender antagonism played second fiddle to rivalries between newer and older views of medical professionalism.

Yet the gender themes in this extraordinary drama remain rich and complex. The trial offers us the spectacle of a woman physician accused of misusing professional power and expertise to manipulate and harm other women. While Dixon-Jones's lawyers employed her sex in her defense, urging that she embraced the "best in femininity" in her work, many detractors found her behavior particularly heinous because she was a woman. As we have seen, contemporary testimony suggests that Dixon-Jones was a classic example of what today would be labeled a "difficult woman"—a woman in authority who is outspoken and perhaps somewhat imperious. Not surprisingly, taking their cues from a number of former patients who spoke to the *Eagle,* several Brooklyn physicians, including Skene himself, accused Dixon-Jones of egregiously poor communication with patients and their families. Many of these, for example, knew only vaguely that there was to be an operation; others were simply told that the doctor would make them well.[36]

Because the concept of informed consent did not exist in this period, and there was a wide range of available opinion on how much information doctors should share with patients before surgery, I read this controversy also as a debate over Dixon-Jones's capacity for empathy—over her ability to treat patients as something other than "clinical material"—and not over whether she violated any formal rules of professional conduct. What is especially intriguing is that her supporters dismissed the idea of close physician-patient communication as either detrimental or unnecessary. A. M. Phelps, surgeon to City Hospital in

New York, testified that he had performed over two hundred laparotomies and had sent many women patients to Jones in Brooklyn. He claimed that it was not usual for physicians to explain to ignorant patients the nature of imminent operations. He himself told them that "they must put themselves in his hands." Charity patients (the "sick poor" who Blackwell worried would be mistreated) were especially problematic because of their ignorance: Phelps believed that these women "might be frightened off the operating table" if they knew too much about what was going to happen to them. As already noted, W. Gill Wylie of Bellevue Hospital confirmed that because laparotomies now had become routine, much less attention was paid to "obtaining consents."[37]

In spite of the support of these colleagues, Dixon-Jones's experimental, active, and manipulative stance toward women's diseases heralded an image of medicine that her Brooklyn colleagues and much of the public were reluctant to accept. Given the prevailing image of the woman physician as nurturing and empathic, Dixon-Jones's being a woman may have actually heightened existing anxieties about the meaning of her various activities for the future of medical practice. Was she not performing aggressive scientific experiments on patients? Using pathological specimens in the name of science to advance her career? Refusing to inform patients properly of her intentions? Surely her conduct was inappropriate for a woman, but lurking below the surface was worry over how representative it was of the entire profession.

Indeed, Elizabeth Blackwell had warned of these developments in a letter to her longtime colleague Mary Putnam Jacobi, a professor at the Post-Graduate Medical School and the Woman's Medical College of the New York Infirmary, and the only woman physician to testify in Dixon-Jones's behalf. Worrying about the recent increase in gynecological surgery and connecting such activity with the horrors of vivisection, Blackwell proposed that Jacobi help her rally women physicians in the United States against unwarranted operative procedures. But Jacobi, like Dixon-Jones, was a woman physician who had embraced advances in technology and research. She gently suggested that Blackwell catch up on her medical reading and think more like a scientist.[38] Moreover, Jacobi added, it would be a terrible mistake to gender new approaches to the cure of disease; women also needed to keep abreast of these developments.[39]

The careers of Elizabeth Blackwell and Mary Dixon-Jones aid us in exploring how representations of gender became embedded in the new ideology of medical professionalism that emerged at the end of the nineteenth century. Elizabeth Blackwell was merely the most eloquent spokesperson for a carefully crafted articulation of female professionalism which, using the language of domesticity, was supremely suspicious of the increasing tendency to treat human beings like objects and of the reductive, activist, and experimental approach of the new breed of ovariotomists. Empathic expertise became an important component of women doctors' public and private image, while motherhood emerged as a central trope of their discourse surrounding the physician-patient relationship. Although the ideology of female professionalism hearkened back to the doctor's traditional role in bedside care, the gendering of professional qualities like empathy was relatively new.

It follows from this that among Dixon-Jones's most virulent critics were other women physicians in Brooklyn who subscribed to a Blackwellian version of female professionalism. In contrast, Mary Dixon-Jones was either oblivious to the subtleties of these behavioral scripts or consciously rejected them. The medicine she practiced—diagnosing and excising diseased organs—evoked a materialist conception of the body that encouraged the practitioner to think, not in terms of the whole patient, but about specific organs and localized infection. Moreover, Dixon-Jones's reference groups were exclusively male; she craved recognition by male colleagues as a surgical innovator of the first rank. Yet in playing the men's game she drew criticism from both sexes for failing to play it with the acceptable demeanor of a woman. In promoting herself, she unwittingly exposed to the scrutiny of investigative journalism unresolved tensions regarding the medical procedures and behavior of the group of specialists to whom she so desperately wished to belong. Those professional tensions, and the gendered language invented in the nineteenth century to give them voice, remain very much with us.

Notes

I am indebted to Barbara Bair, Margaret Finnegan, Louise Newman, Ellen More, Anita Fellman, George Sanchez, Gerald Grob and Tom Cole for helpful readings of this essay.
    1. See Carol Gilligan, *In a Different Voice: Psychological Theory and Women's Development* (Cambridge, Mass.: Harvard University Press, 1982). See also Nel Noddings, *Caring: A Feminine Approach to Ethics and Moral Education* (Berkeley: University of California Press, 1984), and the essays in Janet Finch and Dulcie Groves, eds., *A Labour of Love: Women, Work, and Caring* (London: Routledge & Kegan Paul, 1983), for a sampling of this literature.
    2. Charles Rosenberg, "The Therapeutic Revolution: Medicine, Meaning,

and Social Change in Nineteenth-Century America," in M. Vogel and C. Rosenberg, eds., *The Therapeutic Revolution: Essays on the Social History of American Medicine* (Philadelphia: University of Pennsylvania Press, 1979), 3–25, 10–11.

3. Ibid., 10. See also John Harley Warner, *The Therapeutic Perspective: Medical Practice, Knowledge, and Identity in America, 1820–1885* (Cambridge, Mass.: Harvard University Press, 1986).

4. *Valedictory Address* (Philadelphia: Woman's Medical College of Pennsylvania, 1872), 1–23, esp. 6–7.

5. Warner, *The Therapeutic Perspective*, 235–243.

6. Warner, *The Therapeutic Perspective*, 258; Russell Maulitz, "'Physician versus Bacteriologist': The Ideology of Science in Clinical Medicine," in *The Therapeutic Revolution*, ed. Vogel and Rosenberg, 91–107.

7. See especially Warner's enormously helpful and detailed volume, *The Therapeutic Perspective*.

8. Joan C. Williams, "Domesticity as the Dangerous Supplement of Liberalism," *Journal of Women's History* 2 (Winter 1991):69–88, 71.

9. Erik Erikson, *Childhood and Society* (New York: W. W. Norton and Co., 1950), 267; Blackwell, "The Influence of Women in the Profession of Medicine," in Blackwell, *Essays in Medical Sociology*, 2 vols. (1902; reprint New York: Arno Press, 1972), 1–32, 9–10.

10. Blackwell, "Scientific Method in Biology," in *Essays in Medical Sociology*, 87–150, 126–130.

11. Blackwell, "Influence of Women in the Profession of Medicine," 13; Blackwell, "Erroneous Method in Medical Education," in *Essays in Medical Sociology*, 3–46, 10–12.

12. Blackwell strongly supported clinical casework, postmortem and gross pathology, pathological chemistry, microscopic anatomy and other types of patient-centered investigations. See her "Scientific Method in Biology," in *Essays in Medical Sociology*, 105. Sandra Holton has explored not only Blackwell's thought in this regard but that of other British physicians as well. See Sandra Stanley Holton, " 'Christian Physiology': Science, Religion, and Morality in the Medicine of Elizabeth Blackwell," paper presented at the Pacific Coast Branch of the American Historical Association annual meeting, Kona, Hawaii, August, 1991, and Sandra Holton, "State Pandering, Medical Policing and Prostitution: The Controversy with the Medical Profession Concerning the Contagious Diseases Legislation, 1864–1886," *Research in Law, Deviance, and Social Control* 9 (1988):149–170.

13. Blackwell, "Why Hygienic Congresses Fail," 47–84, 57, 74–75; Blackwell, "Influence of Women in the Profession of Medicine," 12, 19–20, 27–29, in *Essays in Medical Sociology*.

14. As Londa Schiebinger and others have shown, the gendering of certain forms of cognitive thinking had been occurring in scientific discourse since the 1700s. See Schiebinger, *The Mind Has No Sex? Women in the Origins of Modern Science* (Cambridge, Mass.: Harvard University Press, 1989).

15. See Regina Morantz-Sanchez, "Feminist Theory and Historical Prac-

tice: Rereading Elizabeth Blackwell," *History and Theory*, Beiheft 31, (December 1992), for a more extensive analysis of Blackwell.

16. Gulielma Fell Alsop, *History of the Woman's Medical College of Pennsylvania* (Philadelphia: Lippincott, 1950), 109.

17. Deborah Kuhn McGregor, *Sexual Surgery and the Origins of Gynecology: J. Marion Sims, His Hospital, and His Patients* (New York: Garland Publishing, 1989).

18. See Charles Rosenberg, *The Care of Strangers* (New York: Basic Books, 1987), esp. chaps. 7–8.

19. Quoted in Ornella Moscucci, *The Science of Woman* (New York: Cambridge University Press, 1990), 101.

20. Mary Dixon-Jones, "A Case of Tait's Operation," *American Journal of Obstetrics* 17 (November 1884):1154–1161, 1156. The diagnosis of reflex irritation referred to the commonly held view of many gynecologists that diseased reproductive organs could be manifested by a psychological response, in this case, hysteria.

21. Mary Dixon-Jones, "Personal Experiences in Laparotomy," *Medical Record* 52 (August 1897), 182–192, 191.

22. See Howard Kelly and Walter Burrage, *American Medical Biographies* (Baltimore: Normon, Remington Co., 1920), 513.

23. Howard A. Kelly and Walter L. Burrage, *Dictionary of American Medical Biography* (Boston: Milford House, 1971), 677.

24. See Dixon-Jones, "Oophorectomy and Diseases of the Nervous System," *Woman's Medical Journal* 4 (January 1895):1–11, 5; Dixon-Jones, "Removal of the Uterine Appendages—Recovery," *Medical Record* 27 (April 1885):399–402, 400; For Tait's reference to one of Dixon-Jones's articles, see "A Discussion of the General Principles Involved in the Operation of Removal of the Uterine Appendages," *New York Medical Journal* 44 (November 1886):561–567. On Tait, see Jane Sewall, "Bountiful Bodies: Spencer Wells, Lawson Tait, and the Birth of British Gynecology" (Ph.D. dissertation, Johns Hopkins University, 1991).

25. Council Minutes, April 9, May 14, 1884, Kings County Medical Society Archives. A spokesperson for the society told the *Eagle's* reporter in 1889 that her application had been rejected four times for "unprofessional conduct." Brooklyn *Eagle*, May 4, 1889. But there is no evidence of this in the minutes.

26. Brooklyn *Eagle*, February 10, 1892.

27. Pease to Dean Clara Marshall of the Woman's Medical College of Pennsylvania, January 18, 1892, Marshall MSS, Medical College of Pennsylvania; Brooklyn *Eagle*, February 9, 1892; Mosher to Blackwell, November 3, 1883. Mosher MSS, Bentley Library, University of Michigan.

28. Brooklyn *Eagle*, February 9, 1892. See also *Eagle's* comments regarding Jones' unruliness as a witness, her habit of making comments under her breath, and the testimony of Cornelia Plummer, February 4 and February 6.

29. Kelly and Burrage, *Dictionary of American Medical Biography*, 677.

Howard A. Kelly was a distinguished surgeon at Johns Hopkins in the 1890s.

30. Sewall, "Bountiful Bodies," 44. This discussion is indebted to chapter 2 of Sewall's dissertation.

31. I am indebted to Barbara Bair for this insight.

32. Brooklyn *Eagle*, February 19, 1892.

33. Ibid., March 9, 1892. It is important to note that a similar controversy over too much gynecological surgery, which pitted followers of Lawson Tait against followers of Spencer Wells, occurred in Great Britain in 1886 in Liverpool. Dr. Francis Imlach was criticized by the senior surgeon at his hospital and the professor of midwifery at the Liverpool Medical Institution for "unsexing women" and not properly informing ovariotomy patients of the consequences. Imlach ultimately was denied reappointment. See Moscucci, *The Science of Woman,* 160–164.

34. *Eagle,* March 8, 9, February 27, 1892.

35. Apropos of their feelings about Dixon-Jones, consider the following. When the Brooklyn *Eagle* first ran its series on Jones in 1889, the New York Pathological Society appointed a committee to investigate the accusations. The committee did a thorough job, soliciting corroborative letters from a number of people mentioned in the articles, clipping newspaper reports, corresponding with Jones, her son Charles, and the rest of the hospital's trustees. Although the committee concluded that there was not sufficient evidence to censure Dixon-Jones, a member in good standing, we find this curious note from the society's treasurer to the chairperson of the investigating committee: "Dear Doctor . . . Dr. Mary Dixon Jones' dues are *fully* paid up . . . you don't get Mary on the Hip in that way . . . women doctors are a nuisance." May 13, 1889, New York Pathological Society Minutes, New York Academy of Medicine.

36. Brooklyn *Eagle*, February 12, 13, 15, 19, 1892.

37. Ibid., March 8, 9, February 27, 1892. See Kenneth De Ville, *Medical Malpractice in Nineteenth-Century America* (New York: New York University Press, 1990); James Mohr, *Doctors and the Law* (New York: Oxford University Press, 1993).

38. Mary Putnam Jacobi to Elizabeth Blackwell, December 25, 1888. Blackwell Papers, Library of Congress.

39. For more on Jacobi, see Regina Morantz-Sanchez, *Sympathy and Science: Women Physicians in American Medicine* (New York: Oxford University Press, 1985), chap. 7.

SUSAN E. LEDERER

Moral Sensibility and Medical Science
Gender, Animal Experimentation, and the Doctor-Patient Relationship

"When the surgeon finds it necessary to inflict pain,—to cut out a tumor or to amputate a limb to save life,—is it to be said that he is 'cruel,' and that he feels not the human sentiment of pity and sympathy?" asked F. E. Daniel in his 1905 presidential address to the State Medical Association of Texas.[1] At the turn of the twentieth century, the issue of a physician's moral sensibilities, the feelings of pity and sympathy for a suffering patient, drew increasing attention in the heated controversy over animal experimentation. Although calls for physicians to feel more emotional involvement with their patients dated from mid-century, the controversy over vivisection, the nineteenth-century term for any experiment on a living animal, intensified discussions about the nature of the physician's emotional investment in the patient's experience.[2]

Gender was an essential feature of these discussions of medical moral sensibility and the nature of professional distance in the doctor-patient relationship. Both women antivivisectionists and their critics linked the high level of female participation in the animal protection movement to feminine capacities for sympathy and sentiment. But whereas antivivisectionists privileged the heart, some medical critics of the movement pathologized the concern for animal suffering. The feminization of "sympathy" for animal suffering left defenders of animal experimentation groping for a vocabulary to express the scientist's concern for animal and human welfare. "The sufferings of the poor dumb brutes is pictured so vividly as to horrify the reader and awaken sentiments of disgust for the heartless scientist who would dissect a living sentient creature. Is it not to be supposed," insisted F. E. Daniel, "that these investigators have hearts in their bosoms, and deplore that it is necessary? men whose every heart-throb is for humanity, and who do these things, not that they do not love all of God's creatures, and sympathize with their sufferings, but because they love their fellow man more."[3]

The intersections of gender, medical science, and moral sensibility in the controversy over animal experimentation informed turn-of-the-century debates over the physician's ability to retain sensitivity to an animal's suffering and, by extension, to the patient's experience.

In the late nineteenth century animal experimentation was the principal methodology for physicians seeking to reconstitute therapeutic practice on the basis of experimental knowledge. Although practiced by only a small number of investigators, vivisection offered a convenient target for both professionals and laypersons suspicious of the ambitious program to reorient medical therapeutics.[4] Together with the new sciences of bacteriology and immunology, the increasingly reductionist shift in medical epistemology had important implications for the doctor-patient relationship, as physicians drew on information and observations no longer accessible to the sick and their families.

Most Americans welcomed the advances in the medical sciences, but some expressed concern about the affective capacities of the new scientifically trained physician. Despite satisfaction with the therapeutic strides that avoided the "scars of blood letting which depleted the veins of a former generation," former president Grover Cleveland spoke for "the great army of patients" when he insisted that physicians should retain the nonscientific qualities essential to a patient's emotional well-being. "We do not like to think of our doctors as veiled prophets or mysterious attendants," Cleveland observed in 1906, "shut out from all sick-bed comradeship except such as comes through cold professional ministrations, and irresponsive to our need of sympathetic assurance."[5] Scientific information about the etiology of infectious disease, Cleveland explained, did not lessen the patient's need for reassurance in the therapeutic encounter.

The reconstitution of medical science altered the training and practice of physicians. Negotiating the appropriate emotional investment in patients remained a necessary element of professional socialization and identity. The challenge for medical students, William Osler remarked in 1889, was to cultivate a "judicious measure of obtuseness as will enable you to meet the exigencies of practice with firmness and courage, without," at the same time hardening 'the human heart by which we live.'"[6] That many people considered physicians "hardened" by their experiences with the sick, some medical writers conceded, was a problem for the profession. In his enormously popular guide to success in the "nonscientific aspects" of medical practice, the physician D. W. Cathell explained that no working physician could devote his entire energies to the patient's afflictions and sufferings. "If he did," Cathell observed, "the endless chain of misery with which he is brought in contact would prove to be too great a strain on his mind and body, and, through over-care and nerve-strain, would soon unfit him for practice."[7] Despite such difficulties, a doctor's reputation would suffer if he or she failed to manifest "humane anxiety and interest" in a patient.[8] Cathell advised physicians to simulate concern; the surgeon David Cheever, however, objected that the common appearance of indifference among surgeons and physicians often masked an acute sensitivity to the suffering of human patients. "Would that this callousness did more generally prevail," wrote Cheever, and thus lessen the emotional burdens of the surgeon.[9]

Other observers accepted the inevitability, even the desirability, of blunting the sentiments of physicians. Although human dissection desensitized medical students, some argued, the knowledge gained was so important to medical practice that it could not reasonably be sacrificed. "It is true enough that the human body in its wretched nakedness is subjected on the dissection table to most undignified treatment, which is liable to make the student vulgar and rude"; noted the journalist Paul Carus, "but for that reason we cannot abandon dissection."[10] Rather than relinquish dissection, Carus recommended that medical educators strengthen the moral resolve of medical students through prayer and other means. The psychologist James Rowland Angell made a similar argument for animal experimentation. "A loss of original squeamishness" after repeated experiments on animals, Angell argued, might confer a practical benefit to animal subjects, by ensuring "a steadier and prompter hand, with a corresponding decrease in the length of time occupied by the operation and in increased chance of a favorable outcome."[11]

The possibility of even a limited desensitization of physicians as a result of their medical training or practice was unacceptable to American antivivisectionists. The brutalization of physicians assumed enormous importance for these radical critics of animal experimentation. A paramount objection to unrestrained animal experimentation was the deleterious effect on children and adults of deliberate cruelty to animals. The idea that cruelty to animals in childhood led to cruelty to human beings in adulthood had an ancient pedigree.[12] In the nineteenth century, belief in the consequences of cruelty to animals for human beings persisted in suspicion of the moral capability of butchers and fears about experimenting doctors. American antivivisectionists pointed to laws in Pennsylvania and Connecticut that forbade butchers to serve on juries deciding capital offenses, for example, and warned that like butchers, surgeons were liable to lose the finer instincts.[13]

Most antivivisectionists accepted without question the supposedly demoralizing effects of animal experimentation on medical students and physicians. They quoted with approval the warning of a Harvard professor of surgery. "Watch the students at a vivisection," cautioned Henry Jacob Bigelow in 1871, "it is the blood and suffering not the science that rivets their breathless attention. If hospital service makes young students less tender of suffering, then vivisection deadens their humanity and begets indifference to it."[14] Antivivisectionists cited reports of "human vivisection," nontherapeutic experiments performed on human beings, as evidence of the scientific demoralization of the medical profession.[15]

Animal protectionists warned that the vulnerable—the poor, the hospitalized, children, women, and the insane—were especially at risk from vivisecting doctors. The pioneering woman physician Elizabeth Blackwell, whose opposition to animal experimentation reflected her suspicion of the new medical reductionism of the late nineteenth century, explicitly correlated the increase in gynecological surgery with the advent of animal experimentation.[16] "Vivisection tends to make us less scrupulous in our treatment of the sick and helpless poor," Blackwell argued. "It increases that disposition to regard the poor as 'clinical material,' which has become, alas! not without reason, a widespread reproach to many of the young members of our most honourable and merciful profession."[17] Her attacks on the vogue of ovariotomy reflected Blackwell's persistent concerns about the transformation of poor women into "clinical material" for surgeons.[18]

The role of gender in the controversy over sexual surgery and antivivisection in Victorian England has received considerable attention from feminist historians. Some have argued that the fear and anger over sexual surgery and victimization were projected onto the dogs and cats strapped to the vivisector's table. "To protest against vivisection was to challenge a world of male sexual authority and obscenity which they [women] sensed unconsciously, even if they had no direct experience of it," argues Coral Lansbury.[19]

Sexual victimization was not the exclusive motivation for female recruitment into the antivivisection movement. The women who swelled the ranks of American antivivisection societies embraced a maternal responsibility for molding moral development. Just as women entered the political arena in support of temperance as part of their ideological commitment to a nurturant domesticity, antivivisectionists campaigned for animal protection because of their entrenched belief in the demoralizing effects of cruelty to animals and their conviction that as women and mothers they could prevent it. Indeed the American antivivisection movement cannot be understood independently of the massive investment in humane education and the concern about the effects of cruelty to animals on the impressionable minds of children, medical students, and society.[20] The agitation over dissection in the public schools amply illustrates the moral maternalism that animated many antivivisectionists.

In the 1890s the introduction of animal dissection and vivisection in American public schools ignited considerable public discussion. The prominent journalist Agnes Repplier observed that even "conservative" parents were unnerved by the new lessons in physiology. "A cat and a jack-knife do not commend themselves pleasantly as affording a healthy spectacle for children's eyes," Repplier noted, "and there is always a painful possibility that other lessons, not intended, may be taught by this advanced method of illustration."[21] The American Humane Association's 1895 report on dissection and vivisection in American schools declared that most educated Americans did not support animal experimentation in front of schoolchildren.[22] They preferred the use of colored charts and mannequins, which conveyed the rudiments of physiology and hygiene without endangering the moral development of children.[23] The only legislative successes achieved by antivivisectionists in this period involved legal restrictions on vivisection and dissection in public schools. In 1894 Massachusetts enacted a law banning vivisectional demonstrations in elementary and secondary schools. Three years later, the Washington state legislature passed a bill outlawing vivisection in all schools and colleges in the state except for medical and dental schools.[24] In 1919 Maine legislators adopted a bill providing that "No person in any of the schools supported wholly or in part by public money, shall practice vivisection or perform any experiment upon a living animal, or exhibit to any pupil in such school an animal which has been vivisected or experimented upon."[25] By 1922 Alabama, Illinois, Michigan, Oklahoma, Pennsylvania, and South Dakota had statutes banning the exhibition of vivisected animals in public schools.[26]

Opposition to dissection in the schools received a powerful boost from the Woman's Christian Temperance Union (WCTU), which actively supported humane education for children. In 1890 the WCTU formally adopted a Department of Mercy as one of its divisions. This development reflected the broad involvement in moral education championed by the group's dynamic leader, Frances Willard, as well as the belief that intemperance and cruelty were closely related.[27] Like her mentor Mary H. Hunt, the powerful superintendent of the WCTU's Department of Scientific Temperance Instruction, Mary Lovell, the national superintendent of the Department of Mercy, pressed for state

laws to establish humane education in public schools. By 1906 twelve
states had adopted laws requiring humane education in public education.[28]

The WCTU fostered the promotion of humane education through the
organization of Bands of Mercy, groups in which schoolchildren pledged
to be kind to animals. Patterned after English bands of mercy, the first
groups were introduced into the United States by George T. Angell, the
leader of the Massachusetts SPCA.[29] Humane leaders claimed massive
levels of participation in these groups. Lovell reported in 1899 that
nearly 14,000 boys in public schools in Philadelphia alone were enrolled in Bands of Mercy.[30] By 1923 over 140,000 Bands of Mercy in the
United States claimed more than 4 million child members.[31]

Boys were believed to be in special need of moral instruction and
lessons in kindness. Middle-class boys, the historian E. Anthony
Rotundo contends, "were downright lethal to small animals."[32] Many
antivivisectionists regarded male scientists as "little boys who never
grew up." As children, it was said, such boys took delight in disassem-
bling their toys; as adults, they dismembered sentient animals with the
same mindless glee.[33] "The average boy will kill without thought or
regret. This may not be the fault of the boy, but because, perhaps,
nature did not give him the tender heart," Mrs. Fairchild-Allen of the
Illinois Anti-Vivisection Society observed. The failure of nature to in-
still tenderness in boys required parents and teachers "to create a new
heart" in young men. Prison statistics from France and America,
Fairchild-Allen argued, demonstrated that a large proportion of the
male inmates of jails and penitentiaries had never received instruction
in kindness to animals and had lacked pets during their childhood.[34]

The Bands of Mercy movement exerted considerable influence on
organized child activities in the United States. The Salvation Army
modeled its bands of love, in which children pledged to love animals
and to be kind to them, on the bands of mercy. The Boy Scouts also
adopted kindness to animals as one of the obligations of scouthood.[35]
In the second decade of the twentieth century Boy Scouts could earn a
merit badge in first aid to animals. In order to qualify, scouts not only
had to demonstrate an ability to treat domestic and farm animals but
were required to know how to aid a horse in harness when the animal
fell on the street and what to do when animals were being cruelly
mistreated.[36] Although these groups varied enormously in their anti-
cruelty activities, the transient quality of participation should not obscure the ideological commitment on the part of educators, teachers,
and humane advocates to the idea that childhood lessons in kindness
to animals promised great benefit.

At the same time that women antivivisectionists celebrated the moral superiority and capacity for sentiment of their sex, their critics capitalized on the negative associations of female emotionality and impulsivity in the controversy over animal experimentation. From the start, the high level of female participation in the antivivisection movement was used to undermine lay opposition to animal experimentation. For some male physicians, female investment in animal protection represented a natural faculty gone astray. "Sentiment is admittedly the province of women," one physician noted, "but these women are wildly gone off after false gods."[37] Some physicians identified the concern for animal suffering as a species of female psychopathology.

By all accounts, the contemporary assessments of the high level of female participation in the antivivisection movement are reliable. Like their British counterparts, American women quickly assumed the leadership of antivivisection societies. Perhaps the most influential antivivisectionist in the United States was Caroline Earle White, who helped organize the Pennsylvania Society for the Prevention of Cruelty to Animals in 1867. The daughter of the Quaker abolitionist Thomas Earle, White enlisted the support of affluent Philadelphians in the cause of animal welfare. In 1883, spurred by the charismatic leader of the British antivivisection movement Frances Power Cobbe, White organized the American Anti-Vivisection Society to abolish the use of animals in medical research. In addition to her service as the corresponding secretary of the society, White edited the society's monthly magazine, the *Journal of Zoophily*, for over two decades.[38] Although several officers of the American Anti-Vivisection Society were male physicians, including Hiram Corson, reputedly the oldest practicing physician in the United States at the time (and an early champion of women physicians), the society also engaged a woman physician, Amanda M. Hale, to deliver public lectures against animal experimentation. A graduate of the Woman's Medical College of Chicago, Hale was inspired by Elizabeth Blackwell's example to oppose animal experimentation.[39]

The membership of antivivisection societies was largely female. Although men appeared on the boards of directors and in the lists of honorary vice-presidents, women far outnumbered men in the membership rolls. The American Anti-Vivisection Society in 1927, for example, listed 661 active and associated members, including 526 women (79.5 percent) and 132 men (19.9 percent).[40] For many societies, women provided the funds necessary to sustain the crusade against animal experimentation. Female testators, for example, left forty-one of the forty-four legacies (ranging in value from $25 to $10,200) received by the New England Anti-Vivisection Society in the years 1898–1935.[41]

The prominence of women in the controversy over animal experimentation drew negative comment almost from the start. Press reports of ladies attending antivivisectionist meetings dressed in furs and "murderous millinery" (hats adorned with feathers or birds) appeared frequently in both the popular and the medical press. Although some women doubtless did attend antivivisectionist or animal protection meetings in animal skins and aigrette plumes, these reports did not take into account the efforts to persuade women to forgo such ornamentation in their dress. Caroline Earle White characteristically admonished the editor of a Maine medical journal for his reckless sentences about meetings of the SPCA at which "the hat of almost every lady present tells the story of the death agony of from one to six, handsome, useful birds."[42] White supported efforts to discontinue the use of birds or any part of their plumage in women's attire, and joined a new society organized for the purpose of abolishing the wearing of birds or bird feathers. The American Anti-Vivisection Society also sponsored a humane alternative to animal skins, a synthetic fur substitute called "humanifur," to wean women from cruelty in dress.[43]

In addition to efforts to protect birds and fur-bearing animals, antivivisectionists devoted considerable energy to the welfare of food animals. White, for example, considered her most important achievement to be the institution of protective laws in the transportation of cattle by rail. In the 1870s when the investigations of humane society agents revealed that cattle were routinely shipped in closely packed railroad cars without food or water for as long as seventy-two hours, White and her colleagues petitioned Congress for a law requiring that cattle be watered at least once every twenty-eight hours. The Women's Branch of the SPCA, for example, brought a series of complaints against the railroads for violations of the act, and stoutly resisted the attempts of cattlemen to revise the twenty-eight hour rule to forty hours.[44]

These efforts earned little respect from critics of the antivivisection movement, who viewed female commitment to the movement as a product of the fanaticism of "the hysterical and super-sentimental" in whom reason had been neglected. Emotional investment in antivivisection offered yet another reason to withhold the right to vote from women. The impulsivity of women and their undisciplined compassion led some observers to warn that "gusts of unreasoning, uncalculating, hysterical emotion" made woman suffrage a dangerous proposition.[45] To the chagrin of antivivisectionists, the feminist Elizabeth Cady Stanton suggested that the "hysterical force in favor of prohibition, a Puritan Sabbath, *anti-vivisection,* and religion in the United

States Constitution" helped to explain male hesitation about extending the vote to women.[46]

Antivivisection's appeal to women prompted further speculation. Some medical defenders of animal experimentation viewed commitment to antivivisection as a special, feminine form of mental illness. James Warbasse, a New York physician, warned in 1910 that the exaggerated sympathy for dogs on the part of women was actually a manifestation of a "zoophilic psychosis":

> "Antivivisectionists" interest themselves not so much in experiments upon fishes, insects, pigeons, rats, mice, snakes, nor in cruelties to men, cattle, chickens, and sheep. Their interests are bent towards those useless animals which can be made the objects of fondling and which compared with other animals play a minor role in the great field of scientific experimentation.

Explaining that a German researcher had divided women into two types, "the mother-class and the prostitute-type," Warbasse warned that women with an excessive attachment for fondling dogs did not belong to the "mother-type."[47]

This medicalization of love for dogs alarmed some defenders of medical researchers because of the potential backlash from outraged (and unabashed) animal lovers. More typically, the medical defenders of animal experimentation interpreted female investment in antivivisection as a response to maternal deprivation. "The anti-vivisectionists are, for the most part, unmarried or sterile old women whose maternal affections have been centered on animals instead of babies," John R. Murlin informed a New York State assemblyman in 1934.[48] The lack of an appropriate object of female love and compassion served to explain a fixation on animals. Such explanations were not limited to female antivivisectionists; in 1921 a writer in the *Illinois Medical Journal* similarly identified the women who supported legislation to improve maternal and infant health as "endocrine perverts" and "derailed menopausics."[49]

Unflattering depictions of female antivivisectionists also appeared in popular fiction. In Sinclair Lewis's 1925 novel *Arrowsmith,* one unanticipated highlight of the Nautilus Health Fair was the fight between the "anti-nicotine lady" from Chicago, who demonstrated the evils of tobacco every half hour by killing mice with inoculations of cigarette paper, and the "anti-vivisectionist lady," also from Chicago. After branding her opponent "a murderer, a wretch, and an atheist," the antivivisectionist informed her that she was also no scientist. In response the "anti-nicotine lady leaped from her platform, dug her fingers into the anti-vivisectionist lady's hair, and observed with distinctness, 'I'll show you whether I know anything about science!'"[50] Reviewing Lewis's book, one antivivisectionist ruefully observed that the movement owed a debt of gratitude to the "inimitable" George Bernard Shaw "for saving us from unvarying misrepresentation as ignorant and preferably female sentimentalists."[51]

Construing female involvement in antivivisection as the outcome of undisciplined compassion proved a remarkably durable practice in the first half of the twentieth century.[52] Some historians of medicine echoed the explanations of female interest in antivivisection offered by contemporary male medical observers. In a 1954 biography of William Henry Welch, Donald Fleming, for example, described the antivivisection movement as:

> a world alliance of overlapping animal lovers, vegetarians, anti-Listerians, antibacteriologists, and anti-inoculationists; soft muddle-headed women, cold-blooded Amazons and publicity seekers of both sexes, bluff advocates of the old-fashioned godliness and soap-and-water but not carbolic-acid cleanliness, maudlin religionists not averse to blasphemy, medical sectaries, and academic and professional cast-offs—all engaged in a travesty of the intellectual life, snooping about laboratories and ransacking the pages of scientific journals for ammunition.[53]

Male participation in the antivivisection movement required other explanations. In his 1964 history of the Rockefeller Institute, the physician-historian George W. Corner observed that the prominent actor George Arliss lent his name to the antivivisection movement because "the warm-hearted, impulsive people of the stage have always been readily swayed by sentimental appeals."[54] Here and elsewhere emotional lability helped to account for interest in animal protection.

Contemporary critics suggested other motives for male participation in the movement. In 1938, when California animal protectionists garnered the necessary 187,000 signatures for a ballot initiative to prohibit the release of pound animals to medical laboratories, the Stanford University student newspaper reported that support for the bill came from "middle-aged ladies, disappointed in love, and retired businessmen who once read [an Albert Payson] Terhune dog-story."[55] In this case, men appeared as supporters for the antivivisectionist cause, but like childless women, they were individuals with time on their hands and therefore lacking the appropriate object for their energies.

Implicit in some of the characterizations of male antivivisectionists was the idea that concern for animal welfare was not a normal masculine trait. Even though William Randolph Hearst displayed a lifelong interest in animal welfare, his support for antivivisection has often been construed as accommodation to some feminine influence, whether that of his mother, the philanthropist Phoebe Apperson Hearst; his mistress, the actress Marion Davies; or a friend, the dancer Irene Castle.[56] In his biography of the publisher, W. A. Swanberg chronicled Hearst's interest and concern for most animals (Hearst made an exception in the case of rats). "Anyone hurt within his immediate ken, be it human or animal," Swanberg observed, "enlisted his sympathy to such an extravagant degree that he seemed womanly and even ridiculous." Swanberg provided at least one example of this "womanly extravagance"; when Hearst's beloved dachshund Helena died, the publisher wept and ordered her buried beneath a stone inscribed with the legend, "Here lies dearest Helena—my dearest friend."[57] Hearst's outburst over the loss of a pet was viewed as anomalous or eccentric because such emotionality was thought more characteristically female than male.

In 1933 Morris Fishbein, editor of the *Journal of the American Medical Association,* criticized the "ladies and lawyers" whose crusade against animal experimentation required annual legislative appearances from university presidents, professors, physicians, and representatives of industry "to overcome the deluge of misguided sentiment."[58] Idleness and ignorance, Fishbein implied, helped to explain female involvement in the movement. The men who subscribed to laboratory animal protection were less motivated by sentiment or concern for animals than by money. Fishbein suggested that male attorneys and secretaries pursued the antivivisection cause because of their salaries. In the 1940s, as the increase in war-related research intensified the chronic shortage of dogs for experimentation, some medical critics of the "antivivisection racket" argued that men participated in the antivivisection movement to enjoy "unearned power and public notice." These male "faddists of pathological mentality" played on the sympathies of the emotional women who funded the antivivisection societies, feeding them "preposterous pap" and other "dangerous nonsense."[59]

In the 1930s Annie Riley Hale, a writer sympathetic to the antivivisection and antivaccination movements, explicitly addressed the gender implications of the identification of antivivisectionists as hysterical women or effeminate men. Conceding that some of the opposition to vivisection did come from "lonely women in whom frustrated instincts may have produced what modern psychologists term an 'animal neurosis,'" Hale argued that not all interest in antivivisection was emotional: "I have never felt any strong personal attachment for animals, and never in my life had an animal pet of any kind. As a child I preferred dolls, and when I grew older I preferred children as play-

things. My interest in animal life has been intellectual rather than sentimental."[60] In order to refute the "neurotic-women argument," Hale
offered a list of the distinguished men who had opposed vivisection,
including such men of letters as Robert Louis Stevenson, George Bernard Shaw, Mark Twain, William Dean Howells, and Tolstoy. Antici-
pating complaints that literary personalities, perhaps "even though
masculine, are too tame and pallid by nature to make them competent
judges of this red-blooded, two-fisted business of torturing animals,"
she also listed the names of statesmen, naturalists, and jurists, men
whose professional lives suffered no similar imputation of emotional
instability and questionable masculinity.[61]

The controversy over animal experimentation in the first half of the
twentieth century escalated the separation of moral sentiment, or sympathy, and medical science. The feminization of "sympathetic" concern
for animal suffering by both antivivisectionists and their critics diminished the ability to discuss male qualities of caring. But caring remained
essential to the professional identity of physicians—both male and female. What was lacking was an appropriately scientific vocabulary to
contain it.

Notes

1. F. E. Daniel, "Sentiment and Science," *Texas Medical Journal* 20
(1905):429–450.

2. Martin S. Pernick, "The Calculus of Suffering in 19th-Century Surgery," *Hastings Center Report* 13 (1983):26–36.

3. Daniel, "Sentiment and Science," 434.

4. John Harley Warner, *The Therapeutic Perspective: Medical Practice, Knowledge, and Identity in America, 1820–1885* (Cambridge, Mass.: Harvard University Press, 1986).

5. Grover Cleveland, "The Plea of the Patient," *Albany Medical Annals*
27 (1906):153–160.

6. William Osler, *Aequanimitas*, 3rd ed. (Philadelphia: Blakiston Co., 1932),
5.

7. D. W. Cathell and W. T. Cathell, *Book on The Physician Himself and
Things That Concern His Reputation and Success*, 20th cent. ed. (Philadelphia:
F. A. Davis Co., 1906), 71.

8. Ibid.

9. David W. Cheever, "Surgical Morals," *Boston Medical and Surgical
Journal* 134 (1896):281–282.

10. Paul Carus, "The Immorality of the Anti-Vivisection Movement," *Open
Court* 11 (1897):370–376.

11. James Rowland Angell, "The Ethics of Animal Experimentation,"
JAMA 54 (1910):201–203.

12. Keith Thomas, *Man and the Natural World* (New York: Pantheon Books, 1983).

13. See Lloyd G. Stevenson, "On the Supposed Exclusion of Butchers and Surgeons from Jury Duty," *J. Hist. Med.* 8 (1954):235–238.

14. Henry Jacob Bigelow, quoted in Albert Leffingwell, "The Great Protestant against Vivisection Cruelty," *An Ethical Problem*, 2nd ed. rev. (London: G. Bell and Sons, 1916), 117.

15. Susan E. Lederer, *Subjected to Science: Human Experimentation in America before the Second World War*, (Baltimore: Johns Hopkins University Press, 1995).

16. Regina Morantz-Sanchez, *Sympathy and Science: Women Physicians in American Medicine* (New York: Oxford University Press, 1985), 186–191.

17. Elizabeth Blackwell, "Erroneous Method in Medical Education," *Essays in Medical Sociology*, 2 vols. (New York: Arno Press, 1972), 2:43.

18. See the essay by Regina Morantz-Sanchez in this volume.

19. Coral Lansbury, "Gynaecology, Pornography, and the Antivivisection Movement," *Victorian Studies* 28 (1985), 413–437, esp. 422. For a more nuanced view, see Mary Ann Elston, "Women and Anti-Vivisection in Victorian England, 1870–1900," in *Vivisection in Historical Perspective*, ed. Nicolaas A. Rupke (London: Croom Helm, 1987), 259–294.

20. See Judith B. Erickson, "Making King Alcohol Tremble: The Juvenile Work of the Woman's Christian Temperance Union, 1874–1900," *J. Drug Education* 18 (1988):333–352.

21. Agnes Repplier, "Science for Babes," *Anti-Vivisection* 4 (1897):189.

22. American Humane Association, *Report on Vivisection and Dissection in Schools* (Chicago: American Humane Association, 1895).

23. The philosopher William James believed that witnessing a vivisection was not injurious to a normal child, but he still opposed animal experimentation in schools as "wasteful of life and condemnable." American Humane Society, *Report on Vivisection and Dissection in Schools*, 16–17.

24. James Turner, *Reckoning with the Beast* (Baltimore: Johns Hopkins University Press, 1980), 94–95; "Antivivisection for Children," *Medical News*, 67 (1895):181.

25. Howard K. Beale, *Are American Teachers Free?* (New York: Charles Scribner's Sons, 1936), 226.

26. William J. Shultz, *The Humane Movement in the United States, 1910–1922* (New York: AMS Press, 1968), 254–256; Norval Emerson Adams, "The Legal Restrictions Concerning the Teaching of Biology," Master of Science thesis, Indiana University, 1930.

27. Ruth Bordin, *Woman and Temperance: The Quest for Power and Liberty, 1873–1900* (New Brunswick, N.J.: Rutgers University Press, 1990), 98, 109.

28. "Mercy," *Union Signal* (November 29, 1906):14. On Mary Hanchett Hunt, see Philip J. Pauly, "The Struggle for Ignorance about Alcohol: American Physiologists, Wilbur Olin Atwater, and the Woman's Christian Temperance Union," *Bull. Hist. Med.* 64 (1990):366–392.

29. Thomas Timmins, *The History of the Founding, Aims, and Growth of the*

American Bands of Mercy (Boston: Massachusetts Society for the Prevention of Cruelty to Animals, n.d.). Caroline Earle White organized Junior Humane Societies in 1874 to train boys in the ways of kindness before the bands of mercy were instituted. See Sydney H. Coleman, *Humane Society Leaders in America* (Albany, N.Y.: American Humane Association, 1924), 182–183.

30. Mary F. Lovell, "Humane Education," *Union Signal* (August 13, 1899):5.

31. Shultz, *Humane Movement*, 130.

32. E. Anthony Rotundo, "Boy Culture: Middle-Class Boyhood in Nineteenth-Century America," in *Meanings for Manhood: Constructions of Masculinity in Victorian America*, ed. Mark C. Carnes and Clyde Griffen (Chicago: University of Chicago Press, 1990), 15–36.

33. For a graphic illustration, see the cartoon "The Little Boy Who Never Grew Up," *Life* 57 (1911):534.

34. Fairchild-Allen, "Don't Allow Boys to Destroy Life," *Anti-Vivisection* 4 (1897):153.

35. David I. Macleod, *Building Character in the American Boy: The Boy Scouts, the YMCA, and Their Forerunners, 1870–1920* (Madison: University of Wisconsin Press, 1983).

36. Shultz, *Humane Movement*, 132.

37. "Special Correspondence—Philadelphia," *British Medical Journal* 1 (1900):876.

38. For White's life, see Turner, *Reckoning with the Beast*, 50–52; "Mrs. C. E. White, Humanitarian, Dies," *Philadelphia Inquirer*, September 8, 1916.

39. Amanda M. Hale, "The Correlated Duties of the Medical Profession and the Humane Public as Regards Vivisection," *Journal of Zoophily* 7 (1898):20–23.

40. Three members were listed with initials so that their sex was unknown to me. *Forty-fifth Annual Report (1927) of the American Anti-Vivisection Society* (Philadelphia: American Anti-Vivisection Society, 1928).

41. *Annual Report, 1935–1936*, New England Anti-Vivisection Society, National Society for Medical Research (NSMR) manuscripts, National Library of Medicine, Bethesda, Maryland, box 15, folder: New England Anti-Vivisection Society, 1929–1937.

42. Caroline E. White, "Punica Fides," *Journal of Zoophily* 8 (1899):56.

43. "Humanifur Exhibit," *The Starry Cross* 37 (1929):134.

44. Sydney Coleman, *Humane Society Leaders In America* (Albany, N.Y.: American Humane Association, 1924), 250–254.

45. "Mr. Lecky on Women as Antivivisectionists," *Boston Medical and Surgical Journal* 135 (1896):150–151.

46. Quoted in "Passing down the Vale under a Cloud," *Anti-Vivisection* 4 (1897):19. Emphasis in original.

47. James Warbasse, *The Conquest of Disease through Animal Experimentation* (New York, 1910), 159–161.

48. See John R. Murlin to Daniel O'Mara, 14 August 1934, Vivisection

Correspondence, George Hoyt Whipple Papers, University of Rochester.

49. "Maternity and Infancy Bill Sponsored by 'Endocrine Perverts' and 'Derailed Menopausics,'" *Illinois Medical Journal* 39 (1921):143.

50. Sinclair Lewis, *Arrowsmith* (New York: Signet Classic, 1980), 241.

51. Beatrice E. Kidd, "Review of 'Martin Arrowsmith,'" *The Starry Cross* 34 (1925):93–94.

52. See, for example, the photographs emphasizing frivolous female antivivisectionists that accompanied "Animal Experimentation," *Life* (October 24, 1938):46–51.

53. Donald Fleming, *William H. Welch and the Rise of Modern Medicine* (Boston: Little, Brown and Co., 1954), 147–148.

54. George W. Corner, *A History of The Rockefeller Institute, 1901–1953: Origins and Growth* (New York: Rockefeller Institute Press, 1964), 85.

55. John Cobbs, "Bull-Session," *Stanford Daily*, 18 October 1938, California Society for the Protection of Medical Research, carton 1, folder: Society Releases, UCSF.

56. See M. B. Visscher, "A Half Century in Science and Society," in *The Excitement and Fascination of Science*, comp. William C. Gibson (Palo Alto, Calif.: Annual Reviews, 1987).

57. W. A. Swanberg, *Citizen Hearst: A Biography of William Randolph Hearst* (New York: Charles Scribner's Sons, 1961), 456.

58. Morris Fishbein, *The Medical Follies* (New York: Boni & Liveright, 1925), 156–157.

59. Norman T. Kirk, "Mice or Men?" *Hygeia* 24 (1946):498–499, 534, 536–537, 540.

60. Annie Riley Hale, *"These Cults"* (New York: National Health Foundation, 1926), 110. For a recent attempt to divorce sentiment from argument for animal welfare, see the philosopher Peter Singer, who insists that he is not interested in animals nor is he "inordinately fond of dogs." Peter Singer, *Animal Liberation*, 2nd ed. (New York: Random House, 1990), ii.

61. Her list included Bismarck, Admiral Dewey, Senators Henry Blair and George Graham Vest, Alfred Russel Wallace, and Luther Burbank; Annie Riley Hale, *The Medical Voodoo* (New York: Gotham House, 1935), 222.

SECTION TWO

Empathy, Ambiguity, and the Problem of Professional Authority

"I Know Just How You Feel"
Empathy and the Problem of Epistemic Authority

Bureaucratic Rationality and the Erasure of Empathy

Empathy, which figures in nostalgic narratives about bygone and putatively more 'connected' eras as a 'natural' human capacity, has fallen
into disfavor in the climate of scientific instrumentality that prevails in
the late twentieth-century Western world. Its status as a lost—and devalued—art is peculiarly significant for feminist theorists and activists,
I shall suggest. For the places where empathy is still, or again, encouraged (and minimally rewarded) are on the softer, outer edges of social
structures and institutions, away from the hard, core practices, where
real work, informed by *real* knowledge, is said to take place. Those
outer edges, in the main, are the places still reserved for women's
traditional activities, informed by their stereotypically 'lesser' skills, of
which empathy counts as one. Scientific—and, derivatively, social scientific—knowledge is *better*, so the prevailing wisdom goes, to the extent that it eschews empathy, with its affective (hence not objective)
tone, and its concern with the irrelevancies of human particularity.

In this essay I engage critically with the epistemologies that foster
this denigration of empathy: epistemologies that have no place for the
quintessentially empathetic declaration "I know just how you feel." I
contend that a society, and any practice within it, that devalues empathy is poorer, in human terms, for so doing. Yet I argue that empathy is
a thoroughly double-edged phenomenon: its expression is not an unqualified good. Hence it is vital that its would-be advocates develop a
self-critical 'politics of empathy,' to keep them as cognizant of its pitfalls as they may be of its promise.

Kathy Ferguson's diagnosis of how late twentieth-century bureaucratic societies smother values of personal connection in their overwhelming veneration of organization and efficiency is instructive. She
writes: "The requirements of depersonalization in bureaucratic relations mean that individuals are isolated from one another and meaningful social interaction is replaced by formal association. . . . The

structures that isolate us ... undermine our sociality; they harm our capacity to take the perspective of others onto our selves and our situation, to imagine alternatives that come from shared experience."[1]

These hegemonic bureaucratic values inhibit the face-to-face relations that are a sine qua non of empathetic caring practices. In consequence, even institutions that profess to look after people's 'needs'—medical care, social welfare, education—are marked by the same absence of empathy that is palpable throughout the social-political-public domains of mass societies.

Ferguson notes, following Michel Foucault, that bureaucracies are sustained by epistemologies "in which individuals are made into objects of study and human activity is defined as in need of organization, regulation, and control." Her epistemological analyses—that is, her analyses of how 'individuals' are known—highlight these societies' reliance upon science and technology, with the "ever-growing armies of experts offering diagnosis and prescription" that these disciplines produce.[2] Such experts count among the principal actors in the bureaucracy's ongoing projects of eliminating uncertainty and decreasing arbitrariness in the received constructions of the social world, while containing and hoarding knowledge within narrowly circumscribed sectors of power and privilege.[3]

The epistemologies that make individuals into *objects* of study, and hence sustain bureaucratic practices, are the epistemologies that produce and inform post-positivist, empiricist social science. In their monologic, unidirectional character, their privileging of a spectator, observational model of evidence gathering, and their assumption that knowledge is produced to facilitate manipulation, prediction, and control, these epistemologies tacitly construct a picture where *empathetic* knowing finds no place. The term is a misnomer; and the activity it purports to name could count, epistemologically, as only a pale, and intermittently occurring precognitive aberration.

In their conviction that knowledge is neutrally given, found, not made, these epistemologies can accord no epistemic worth to the attunement, the sensitivity, that certain kinds of knowing demand; in their separation of reason and emotion, they foreclose possibilities for adequate analyses of emotional knowing: indeed, the very term becomes oxymoronic. In their adherence to a positivistically derived unity-of-science unity-of-knowledge credo, these epistemologies can only know objects that can be analyzed, classified, quantified, as the 'data' of physical science purportedly can: hence they rely on and reproduce an instrumental rationality that translates, in the social-moral context, into an abstract, impartial calculus of means and ends. In the social sciences and the practices they inform, these epistemologies engender structures of epistemic authority in which experts, who allegedly speak 'from nowhere,' stretch and mold the vagaries of human experiences, procrustean-style, into categories of social manageability. Hence a scientifically or medically known client becomes a 'case': and the case, to quote Foucault, is "the individual as he may be described, judged, measured, compared with others . . . it is also the individual who has to be trained or corrected, classified, normalized, excluded, etc."[4] These social sciences produce the experts on whom disciplined and disciplinary societies rely to ensure that populations, patients, and clients remain docile and bureaucratically malleable.

The claim "I know just how you feel" is at the furthest remove from the detached and impersonal knowledge claims that are the focus of standard epistemological analysis. Its *grammar* (in the Wittgensteinian sense[5]) locates it in an exchange that assumes the possibility of engaging experientially, affectively with another person. Most people know what the claim implies: when it 'rings true' it is at once affirmative, comforting, and *consolidating*. It proclaims, however fleetingly, a bond, a sense of mutuality. Politically, the early, sisterhood-affirming consciousness-raising of second-wave feminism produced just such moments. Hence some feminists maintain that the affiliative qualities that some women have tended to develop in Western societies under patriarchy are just the qualities that could transform a world of depersonalized instrumentality into a less alienating place.[6] Elaborations and critiques of this general idea, and of the 'cultural' or 'maternal' feminism that it generates, have figured prominently in the recent work of white anglophone North American feminists. Especially in response to the writings of Carol Gilligan and Nel Noddings, many such analyses have concentrated on the moral-political implications of justice-and/or-care. Within these debates, empathy often figures as a taken-for-granted component of care.

As a point of entry into these questions I am focusing on empathy expressed in an everyday utterance, which relies upon a knowledge claim that contrasts starkly with the disengaged knowledge of bureaucratic institutions. "Knowing just how you feel" is the antithesis of the observational knowledge that makes individuals into objects of study and seeks to achieve impersonal control. The divergence between these modes of knowing highlights the epistemological contrasts that shape the justice and/or care debates; it indicates one direction that projects of developing 'people friendly' epistemologies might take.

The 'justice talk' of utilitarian and contractarian moral theory commonly uses the language of rights; it derives from and sustains conceptions of instrumental rationality.[7] Because it presupposes an on-tology/epistemology of sameness, it need not individuate: each person counts as one interchangeable, impartially assessible unit, paradoxi-cally called 'an individual.' The language of justice and fairness is ad-ministratively smooth, neat. It can sort people and circumstances, match them up, and indicate how rewards and punishments, goods and ser-vices, should be distributed equitably, impartially.[8] It lends itself well to formal epistemological analysis: its claims can be articulated in the standard S-knows-that-p propositional rubric, and verified or falsified accordingly. This is the epistemology that ensures the tidy functioning of mass societies. In contrast with its closed, 'problem-solved' knowl-edge, 'care talk'—that is, the language of care and the practices it in-forms—is most effective when it individuates appropriately. Criteria of appropriateness have always to be negotiated, case by case, and open-endedly. Kathryn Jackson and Owen Flanagan make the point: "Whereas justice as fairness involves seeing others thinly, as worthy of respect purely by virtue of common humanity, morally good caring requires seeing others thickly, as constituted by their particular human face, their particular psychological and social self. It also involves taking seriously, or at least being moved by, one's particular connection to the other."[9] In short, caring depends for its effectiveness upon responsible knowledge of the other: upon finding out who she or he is in the pertinent respects, resisting stereotypes, swift categorizations; upon checking one's conjectures against his or her sense of herself/himself.[10]

The empathy which, for many theorists, is an integral component of good care—is constitutive, in effect, of its cognitive dimension—re-quires, for its successful practice, a radical epistemological shift. Its practitioners will eschew many of the central tenets of the spectator epistemologies that treat persons as objects, to move toward an episte-mological stance for which (as I have argued elsewhere, following Annette Baier), persons are, essentially, 'second persons.'[11] An episte-mological position constructed around 'second person' thinking pre-supposes relationships qualitatively different from those assumed by third-person talk *about* people. 'Second persons' engage with one an-other and care about the quality of that engagement—whether in fond-ness or in fury. A Sartrean constitution of other persons as starkly 'Other,' as *en soi*, shows by contrast what I mean; as does Marilyn Frye's image of the arrogant (masculine) eye, which "gives all things meaning by connecting all things to each other by way of their refer-ences to one point—Man."[12] Imposing meaning on someone else's ex-istence from a position removed from it, or ignorant of and indifferent to its specificities, is at the furthest remove from second person knowing. Impersonal interactions often mask a similar ignorance and indifference, in their disinterested neutrality.

By contrast, empathy at its best resists closure, invites conversation, fosters and requires 'second-person' relations. And empathy, moreover, is a self-reflexive skill. When it is well developed, well practiced, it incorporates a capacity to assess its own aptness: a capacity that enables its practitioners to judge the kind and degree of empathy a situation, a person, or a group requires; and to hold back at places where their habitual empathetic practices may be inappropriate, excessive, or inadequate. Empathy at its best calls for a finely tuned sensitivity both in its cognitive moments (working out how much one can/should know) and in its active ones. And neither 'moment' is self-contained: they are mutually constructive and inhibiting.

Yet empathy-at-its-best is a rare occurrence; nor does empathy count as an unqualified good either in intimate or in wider political contexts. Indeed, current feminist concern with the distribution of speaking positions across social orders, with questions about who can legitimately speak for and about whom, locates theorists who advocate the value of empathy—and I count myself among them—within the terms of a delicate set of tensions. Experientially, in friendships and close relationships, many people would affirm the possibility and desirability of empathy. Feminist critiques of the impersonal structures of mass societies, of which Ferguson's is a salient example, often translate into calls for empathetic engagement. The point seems to be that empathy presupposes and fosters the mutuality on which 'true' or 'authentic' community—if such terms retain any purchase in these postmodern times—must depend. Its cultivation appears, therefore, to be vital to personal and social renewal. Nonetheless, there are reasons for wariness in expressing and responding to empathy: reasons that prompt my claim that empathy is a thoroughly double-edged phenomenon. I shall address some of them before suggesting how empathetic knowing might realize its promise after all.

Who Empathizes? Who Cares?

I have noted that, in the justice and/or care debates, empathy tends to figure as a necessary component of care. The assumption is—and I think it is valid—that without some degree of empathy (by which, here, I mean 'feeling with' another person) adequate, appropriate care cannot be offered. Yet this is the problem: in much of the literature that claims a debt to Nancy Chodorow's work on object relations theory[13] and also in the popular wisdom, empathy figures as a trait, a capacity, that is peculiarly, even "naturally" female. Even where female empathy is represented as a product of historically specific socialization processes, the assumption often is that these processes are well adapted to elicit the latent features of a nature uniquely susceptible to just this kind of molding. Whether in discussions of the survival skills that women develop in situations of truncated power and privilege, or of feminine connectedness contrasted with masculine separateness, the folklore is sustained that women just *are* empathetic. Ferguson notes that "connection with others is a primary given of . . . [most women's] lives . . . ;" that "women's moral judgments are closely tied to feelings of empathy and compassion for others,"[14] with an appeal to women's 'characteristic' experiences as care givers. Although she neither aggregates nor essentializes women, her analysis often implies that there is something natural, or at least quite appropriate, here. Marcia Westkott refers to "women's *need* to affiliate . . . to empathize, to be connected, to relate."[15] Such naturalistic assumptions confound arguments in favor of the politically reconstructive potential of empathetic practices.

My claim is not that naturalistic presuppositions inevitably thwart emancipatory projects. Rather, I am drawing attention to a set of assumptions that they generate about the putative "naturalness" of female reproductive life in general and, derivatively, of female empathic and caring activities.[16] For if empathy is simply natural—simply (to adopt a de Beauvoirean idiom) a manifestation of women's immanence, their species being—then it is impossible to see it as the skilled achievement that it often is. Empathy becomes just another dimension of female reproductive life, a matter of merely doing what comes naturally, hence neither praise- nor blameworthy, nor an accomplishment with any political implications either way. More seriously, as long as the myth of empathy's natural femaleness persists, there is no question of extending its scope beyond a conservatively demarcated female domain. Empathetic values can be cast as primarily parochial, confined to inner circles of personal intimacy.[17] An ethic of care constructed around such an assumption could endorse a self-serving complacency that would make it morally and politically 'good enough' just to empathize with one's 'nearest and dearest,' as most women 'normally' do. There would be little point in suggesting that this is a knowledge-saturated skill, the product of a process of hard work—and that men should work at it too. The idea of empathetic *knowing* becomes meaningless when empathy is conceived as a merely instinctual (therefore neither rational nor valuable) female attribute; and the idea that men should participate is as ludicrous as the suggestion that they take part in breastfeeding.

The folklore that 'feminizes' empathy contrasts oddly with the fact that the term 'empathy' makes a relatively late and an uneasy entry into everyday English. 'Empathy' is a translation of Freud's *Einfühlung*: literally 'in-feeling,' 'feeling into.' (Alix Strachey, one of Freud's translators, claims that Ernest Jones invented it; she calls it "a vile word, elephantine, for a subtle process."[18]) Genealogically, the term is quite interesting. Although it would be intuitively, experientially implausible to suggest that, pre-Freud, empathetic practices, empathetic knowing did not occur, the naming process within professional psychiatry confers a legitimacy and an authority on knowing of this kind that it could not have claimed as a matter-of-course, natural response.

In *The Empathic Imagination*, Alfred Margulies writes of empathy as at once central to the workaday world of a therapist, and riddled with paradox. For him, this is a delicate practice that demands a "creative capacity to suspend closure, to know and not to know simultaneously"; for the self psychology of Freud's successor, Kohut, empathy becomes a capacity "to know via vicarious introspection."[19] David M. Berger describes empathy as an "'emotional' knowing of another human being rather than intellectual understanding," characterizing it as "an essential prerequisite for the psychoanalytic therapist."[20] These descriptions suggest that alongside empathy as a quiescent and undervalued female mode, there is in circulation a positive conception for which (speaking again in the existential idiom) empathy is a *project*-directed, delicate, and respected skill, integral to the practice of highly trained professionals.

It is instructive to compare everyday assumptions about empathy's connection to women's putatively 'natural' care giving with its elevation to a finely tuned professional achievement. My point is not to propose a crude equation between these claims for empathy and the maleness of the claimants. Rather I want to note a continuity here with processes, now well documented in feminist literature, in which the skills and artifacts that inform women's traditional domestic lives (cooking, herbal remedies, old wives' tales, gossip) are judged valueless when they merely emanate from what women do,[21] yet are promoted to the status of scientificity and professional attainment when men 'discover' them. Westkott notes that "men take for granted that women will be caring and empathic, but they implicitly and explicitly devalue women and refuse to reciprocate."[22] By contrast, Margulies compares the empathy of the professional therapist to a poetic understanding that passes through a Husserlian phenomenological reduction to achieve a condition that is "not merely a resonating with the other, but an act of will and creativity."[23] The politics of gender are striking here. Not only is

empathy a devalued female trait—and need—in the folklore of Western societies; but there is an internal tension within the language of
empathy that demeans its quotidian female associations by separating
them from the professional context from which one of its most salient
current meanings derives. As a female practice its knowledgeable, rational dimension disappears into the chaos of inchoate affectivity; as a
male-defined professional accomplishment it is a peculiarly effective,
nuanced mode of knowing.[24]

Therapeutic empathy—whether the therapist is female or male—is
marked from the outset by an asymmetry in the power of its participants. Hence it produces a third tension: the issue of uses and abuses
within the power/knowledge structures that empathy claims establish.
Even so simple and seemingly direct a claim as "I know just how you
feel" is potentially both caring, supportive, affirmative of mutuality
and coercive, intrusive, cooptive. There is no doubt that empathy is
central among the ingredients that make and sustain close friendships:
empathy as expressive as much of joy and pleasure as of sorrow or
pain. If I can never believe that my friend knows how I feel, it is not
easy to see how a friendship can survive. Yet even in personal relationships, centered around warranted assumptions of mutuality, of knowing how things are with one another, such declarations have to be kept
open to reinterpretation. One can always get it wrong; "vicarious introspection" can be trusted only when it finds confirmation, often in ongoing conversation. The 'fit' of each empathetic claim has to be assessed,
separately and sensitively.

The negative, imperialist potential of declared empathy is most evident in situations informed by spectator epistemologies, and marked
by an obvious power differential. Medical consultations can be like
this; but there are many possibilities. Where there is a difference of
power, knowledge, expertise, a claim to 'know just how you feel' can
readily expand into a claim that I will tell you how you feel, and *I* will
be right, even though you might describe it differently, for your perceptions are ill-informed, and my greater expertise must override them.
Monologic, unidirectional epistemologies, where propositional knowledge claims are uttered *by* a 'subject' *about* an 'object' (*S* knows that *p*),
legitimate such moves. In women's confrontations with authoritarian
expertise, such exchanges are common. Moreover, the same sensitivi-
ties and skills that make beneficent empathy possible can be turned to
manipulative and malevolent purposes.

Ferguson notes that, in bureaucratic institutions, both clients and
low-ranking bureaucrats become 'the second sex.' In the social services,
where "the language . . . is . . . invaded by techniques culled from busi-

ness management, social workers are . . . removed from any intimate linguistic or institutional contacts that might serve as the basis of a common identity," while "the client must learn to please . . . to give the required recognition to administrative authority."[25] Clients become 'the second sex,' for they must adopt women's traditional positions of 'otherness' and compliance, together with their survival strategies, simply in order to maneuver within these complex structures; and women who are clients/patients are doubly disempowered. The contestability of privileged access, and the issues of power and authority implicated in its contestation, are the epistemological issues here. Often, in such a context, empathetic declarations produce only a sense of alienation or of forced, false mutuality.

Yet two possible consequences of this line of argument need to be forestalled. I am neither making a case, here, for the inviolability of privileged access claims, nor am I contending that empathy is possible only where there is perfect symmetry of power and expertise. One of the most radical points of departure in a move to 'second person,' dialogic epistemologies is a recognition that—where the knower/known relation can be conceived as a two-person one—*each* participant is a 'second person,' capable of engagement with the other. This point is pertinent to the privileged access issue in the sense that it opens a space for questioning, not just of the extent to which I know how *you* feel, but also of the extent to which you know how you feel, and I know how *I* feel. Privileged access is much less privileged than it was on the old empirical model where knowledge of one's own experiences was upheld as the transparent, immediate, and incontestable basis of all knowledge worthy of the name.

Contesting that privilege creates more, rather than fewer, problems for an analysis of empathy, even as it engages more fully with the subtlety of empathetic knowing. In affluent Western patriarchal societies, one of the most striking cognitive asymmetries has been unequivocally gender-determined: men alone (white, affluent, educated men) could have authoritative knowledge; women, who were more dependent on intuition, feeling, empathy than on reason, could claim minimal cognitive authority. Hence they were not to be believed, even about how they felt, about the deliverances of "their own" experiences.[26] The tension here is peculiarly delicate; for even the most heart-felt expression of how I feel now is open to clarification, discussion, reinterpretation. Those processes might help me to understand my experiences better, even as they enable my interlocutor to know—or to see that she does not/cannot know—how I feel; *or* they might count for me as a gross, a disempowering violation.

These problems notwithstanding, I want to hold open the possibility that empathy at its best can be realized even in situations of asymmetrical power and expertise. Empathy is a rare and a fragile achievement: that I hope to have made clear. But it is not an all-or-nothing occurrence; it admits of degree, and varies situationally. Nor are its possibilities annihilated by power asymmetries; rather, such asymmetries need to be articulated, analyzed, and constantly negotiated. Hence far from being a 'natural' and instinctive happening, empathy, as one examines its nuances, becomes increasingly intricate, tangled, difficult. Its rarity needs to be respected; and there are times where refraining from empathy in favor of a more removed professionalism may be the most empathic course of action. It takes an equivalent sensitivity to recognize those times for what they are, and to respond accordingly.

Interpretation: A Better Way?

It may appear from the stark picture I have drawn of post-positivist social science and the objectivist epistemologies that inform it that I am naming the social sciences, indifferently and indiscriminately, as the cause of the malady I am discussing. I intend, however, to look to recent developments in the social sciences for a way of embarking on a cure. Ferguson claims that the bureaucracy, for all its pervasiveness, is "uneven and incomplete" and hence unable "totally to absorb the field of enquiry."[27] I am suggesting that the same is true of the positivist legacy in the social sciences, for all its hegemonic pretensions.

In her book *Gender and Knowledge: Elements of a Postmodern Feminism,* Susan Hekman suggests that twentieth-century methodological disputes in the social sciences have had a catalytic effect in unsettling some of the fundamental assumptions of positivism. Of particular significance is a new focus on "the interpretive character of all human knowledge"[28] and a sustained (if not wholly achieved) project to unseat the physical sciences from their paradigmatic place. It is clear that the positivist orthodoxy still commands allegiance in academic social science and among practitioners in the public domain. In the universities, graduate students still argue in vain for the opportunity to pursue qualitative research with the blessing of the academy; the bureaucracy shows that there is life in positivism yet. Moreover, it would be folly to discount the effectiveness of positivist-empiricist methods, judiciously deployed, in enabling people to find the information they need to negotiate the everyday circumstances of their lives and hence, too, in order to be appropriately empathetic. My quarrel is with its hegemonic status: with the imperialist reductivism of its assumption that knowledge is nothing more than information; and with its unity-of-science contentions. Hekman, I think, overstates the case in claiming that *all* knowledge is interpretive, implying that positivism and interpretation are dichotomously distinct. In good epistemic practice they will function as mutually supportive instruments. Nonetheless, precisely because of the hegemonic pretensions of positivism, it is useful to examine the promise of interpretation and to be cautiously optimistic in noting that, in the social sciences, the interpretive challenge is increasingly vociferous, claiming an ever larger share of the discursive space.

I want to suggest that an emergent interpretive epistemology has considerable promise for the construction of empathetic knowledge in particular, and more responsible knowledge of human subjects in general, than pre-interpretive social science could afford, especially if such an epistemology preserves a 'realist' commitment from its positivist heritage.[29] I am not claiming that interpretation can supersede positivism and its successors to become the new paradigm, however. Any suggestion that there could be a single paradigm would itself be anti-interpretive, reinstating a will to closure just where interpreters resist most strongly.[30] Interpretive projects are only beginning to establish themselves, both for feminists and elsewhere: it is too soon to determine their status. Moreover, interpretation can also be monologically construed, practiced in an authoritarian—coercive—manner. Interpretation also invokes responsibility requirements, both *to* the 'datum' and *with* the subject whose experience is interpreted. Interpretive enquiry has to work on a case-by-case basis, to resist totalizing or universalizing, to refuse closure. There can be no definitive statement of what it is, 'in the final analysis'; yet projects can be characterized as primarily interpretive, and reasons can be adduced in favor of naming them thus.

With a debt to Gadamerian hermeneutics as one of their principal shaping forces, interpretive methodologies contest the fact/value and reason/emotion splits that are central to orthodox positivism. They focus on particularity, context, texture; they resist monologic, abstract formulations to maintain that meanings—the stuff of which their enquiry is made—are intersubjective, hence irreducible to "individual subjective states, beliefs, or propositions."[31] With their concentration on experiences and constructions of meaning, interpretive approaches resist the formalisms in which subjectivity disappears into a deductive-nomological model; with their commitment to *ongoing* interpretation and reinterpretation, they escape the tyranny of obdurate privileged access claims. Emphasizing the constitutive role of discourse in its dialogic, conversational, and narrative modes, interpretive approaches eschew the spectator tradition for a participant model in which listeners participate as fully as speakers, and neither listener nor speaker position is fixed.

I shall not engage in the debates that interpretive methodologies, in their turn, generate.[32] I want rather to suggest how epistemologists, working within the gaps that positivistic *and* bureaucratic institutional structures leave open, could show that interpretive, empathetic *knowledge* is sometimes possible, and thus could infiltrate pre-interpretive societies to effect significant transformations. With this project in mind, I return to the tensions I discuss in the previous section of this essay.

Hekman's contention that all knowledge is interpretive is especially pertinent to the tension produced by representing empathy as a natural female trait. Indications of how female 'nature' should best be realized and maternal/cultural feminist projects of revaluing women's 'natural' capacities and attributes tend tacitly to subscribe to a belief that nature, at least, is there, given, a fixed point in a sea of flux. Many feminists preserve this belief, for example, in claiming that sex is given, but gender is constructed—that biology is a datum whose uncontaminated reality could be revealed if cultural accretions were stripped away. Yet Michelle Rosaldo notes that appeals to *biology* in search of the natural source of gender assume that biological differences are "really real." She writes: "Relationships, in such accounts, are contracts forged by individuals who are already fully formed. Natural differences are what make us unite, and from such instrumental unions grows society." For Rosaldo, most of the differences commonly designated biological are "no more natural than the claim by Bushmen that women need male partners to light fires and shoot game."[33] (Late twentieth-century Western counterparts of these 'needs' are not difficult to name.) In like vein, Henrietta Moore comments that "the concept of 'mother' is not merely given in natural processes (pregnancy, birth, lactation, nurturance), but is a cultural construction which different societies build up and elaborate in different ways. . . . The concept of 'woman' is constructed through these different constellations of ideas."[34] Here we have no mere labeling of a biologically natural kind. Feminist critics of the politics of biology have demonstrated beyond dispute that biology is as much a construct as it is a given:[35] most would agree that in making it the basis of a moral-political-social law, "we think poorly and inconsistently about biology."[36]

Locating empathy in an untheorized female nature, 'naturally' confined to the caring, nurturing activities of a 'private' domain, robs it of political significance. Working, rather, to determine, case by case, whether any of its points are given, fixed, can begin to reveal the extent

to which female 'nature' is a political construct, a contingent, historically specific way of realizing the biological intractables that do appear
to be relatively stable. Such an inquiry pries open the associations between women, empathy, and caring, to submit all of the terms to analysis. Women's nature, caring, and the social orders in which these are
aligned and denigrated are at once facts and artifacts, open to ongoing
interpretation, genealogical analysis, and deconstruction. An informed
refusal of the naturalistic biases that construct empathy as merely instrumental becomes possible when these intransigent alignments are
forced to shift.

I have noted that the construction of empathy as a therapeutic skill is
equivocally instructive. On the one hand, elaborations of its professional implications convey some sense of its finesse, its delicacy, and its
intelligently sensitive quality. On the other hand, the location of
empathetic knowing in a professional setting produces power asymmetries that can turn this ideally reciprocal, mutually affirming skill
into an imperialistic, coercive practice. Interpretations and reconstruc-
tions have to work within these equivocations.

The idea of 'vicarious introspection' falls on the negative side of the
balance sheet. Its individualistic, monologic tenor places it closer to
such formal analyses as Thomas Nagel's *The Possibility of Altruism* than
to the mutual, reciprocal process that empathy requires. Nagel's project
is "to discover for . . . altruism . . . a basis which depends . . . on formal
aspects of practical reason."[37] Crucial to its completion is a recognition
of the possibility of putting oneself in another person's place, which in
turn requires a recognition of others as persons like oneself. Yet the
formal nature of the discussion limits such recognition to judgments of
abstract, formal sameness: this is a moral position informed by the
epistemology of sameness that informs and regulates justice-talk and
the bureaucracy. Nagel does not question the possibility of concluding,
from a spectator position not unlike the view from nowhere that he has
since developed, that another person is 'like himself'; nor does he worry
about individual differences, social-political-cultural-*gendered* locations,
that might make putting oneself in another's position more an act of
arrogance than of altruism. (As Nancy Holland remarks: "It is only
those who need not take the reality of others seriously, whose lives do
not depend on understanding how others see the world, who can assume that all lives . . . are basically the same—and that very assumption perpetuates their power."[38]) Yet Nagel has no doubt that, formally
at least, any rational, self-conscious agent can act as a vicarious, surro-
gate knower of the circumstances, desires, needs of another person. An
empathy that casts itself as a form of 'vicarious introspection' risks

falling into just these errors. (Consider Robert Hogan's claim that the "disposition to take the moral point of view is closely related to empathy *or role taking*,"[39] and a test he designed to "measure" empathy. 'Subjects' were to rate themselves with respect to the item "As a rule I have little difficulty in 'putting myself into other people's shoes'": for Hogan, this item is notable for its capacity to reveal socialization achievement.)[40]

The pre-interpretive crudity of these approaches—even of Nagel's elegant, formalistic approach—is their most striking feature. They rightly occasion the feminist concerns I refer to above, about who can legitimately speak for and about whom—about the distribution of speaking positions across social orders. These are questions feminist anthropologists have been asking for nearly two decades: their contributions attest to the promise of revisionary, interpretive social science. Moore, for example, writes of a move toward "radically interrogating the assumptions on which anthropological interpretations rest"; noting that in what I call the 'pre-interpretive period,' "Other cultures were . . . a way of understanding, commenting and reflecting on the peculiarity of Western culture. The question was not so much 'What are the other societies of the world like?' but rather 'Is everybody like us?'"[41] Nagel—and Hogan—do not ask; they presume. Just as equations of empathy with 'female nature' leave that nature an uninterpreted given, so these analyses assume the 'givenness' of a stable, infinitely replicated self that can be known observationally, or from the incontestability of its privileged access, first-person utterances.

These hesitations notwithstanding, the more circumspect aspects of Margulies's reading of empathy—including the parallels he draws with a Husserlian 'bracketing' of assumptions—reveal its potential as a mode of knowing that lends itself, analogically, to transformative, politically revisionary elaborations. "Empathy," he cautions, "must be checked and rechecked . . . if one is not to lose one's way and make a fiction of the other." It requires "the capacity to go against the grain of needing to know"; it is inextricably caught in paradox, and moves within it. Yet it is effective as a process in which, at its best, "*each* participant lives vicariously in the other's world," however fleetingly.[42] Here is none of the obliteration of subjectivity that bureaucratic institutions require for their efficient operation. From an interplay of active, engaged subjectivities, insights are achieved: insights that are not primarily *intra*subjective, but *inter*subjective. There may be no closure, but there are points of action, nodal points informed by a developing understanding, testable for its effectiveness. The myth that it is impossible to know or act in the absence of theoretical, methodological rigidity is put in question. These moments of realized possibility may be rare: I could not, in light of my cautionary tone in the previous section, claim perfect optimism, after all, for the possibilities of a ubiquitous empathy to displace the bureaucratic structures of technological society. But I am suggesting that some such practices of interpretation may be the only possible moves, both in personal and in broader ecological-developmental contexts. I am suggesting, further, that it may often be possible to designate places at which strategies of interpretation and narrative can be circulated through policymaking situations and other 'second-personal' encounters, with the aim of opening out and working with the tensions that positivistic epistemology has kept alive.

Ethical-Political Implications

One of the most notable features of these interpretive projects is their preservation of ambiguity—a feature in which they contrast most sharply with the crudity of pre-interpretive epistemologies. Yet in this feature they resonate with the moral-political position Simone de Beauvoir elaborates in *The Ethics of Ambiguity*: a work which, I shall suggest, is a particularly rich resource for understanding the promise of empathy. (Hence it may be no coincidence that Margulies claims a debt to existentialism and existential psychology.) The title of de Beauvoir's work locates it in opposition to the moralities and epistemologies of the bureaucracy: recall Ferguson's reference to its projects of "eliminating uncertainty and decreasing arbitrariness." She contends that bureaucracies "aim at arranging individuals and tasks so as to secure continuity and stability and to *remove ambiguity*."[43] Ambiguity threatens anarchy; it impedes the instrumentality on which the bureaucracy's very existence depends. Yet de Beauvoir constructs an ethical-political position around just this feature: ambiguity.

In the mode of the universal leveler there can be no authentic ethics, de Beauvoir contends: "A collectivist conception of man does not concede a valid existence to such sentiments as love, tenderness, and friendship; the abstract identity of individuals merely authorizes a comradeship between them by means of which each one is likened to each of the others."[44] Her ethics grants pride of place to ambiguity because it is an ethics of particularity: particulars encountered in their specificity evade summing up, stasis, closure. For de Beauvoir, the source of values is not in the world, or in "impersonal, universal man," but in "the plurality of concrete, particular men projecting themselves towards their ends on the basis of situations whose particularity is as radical and irreducible as subjectivity itself."[45] Subjectivity constitutes itself in choices, made in the context of previous and potentially future choices, and *in relations with others*. Readings of de Beauvoir (such as Hekman's[46]) that emphasize the stark individualism that she adopts from Sartre miss the force of her—intermittent—departure from Sartrean thought in her emphasis on responsibility for and with others. According to de Beauvoir, mutual recognition between subjects is not merely possible, it is ethically required.

Attempts to merge one's subjectivity with another, or to subsume the other under one's own perspective (as Nagel risks doing), thwart such recognition. De Beauvoir writes: "It is only as something strange, forbidden, as something free, that the other is revealed as an other. And to love him genuinely is to love him in his otherness and in that freedom by which he escapes."[47] Empathy at its best preserves yet seeks to know the "strangeness," respects the boundaries between self and other that the "forbiddenness" affirms, does not seek to assimilate or obliterate the "freedom." Its ambiguity is manifested in coming to terms simultaneously with the other's likeness to oneself, and her/his irreducible strangeness, otherness.

Epistemologies that make individuals into *objects* of study annihilate these possibilities. When persons are studied, disciplined, classified as objects would be, then the meaning of their existence is vicariously reduced to the contingent givens of their (empirical) facticity.[48] Such a reduction occurs when the practices and survival strategies of an oppressed group are represented as 'natural' facts, and enlisted to explain and justify the social structures that produce them. Appeals to women's natural subservience to the requirements (including the empathy requirements) of species being are the salient examples here. In contrast to the reductivism that perpetuating these moves requires, de Beauvoir affirms: "The ambiguity of freedom . . . introduces a difficult equivocation into relationships with each individual taken one by one."[49] Because de Beauvoirean ambiguity is at once ethical and political, making no forced distinction between the two; because it resists closure yet constantly requires action; because it respects and addresses the others it encounters, it can become a valuable catalyst for developing viable forms of interpretive empathy.

Responsible empathetic knowing will start from a recognition that mutuality can never be assumed, but it can sometimes be realized, not just between two people, but by extending a second-personal mode into ever wider contexts. Public policy discussions that eschew postures of remote expertise to engage directly with the people who will be affected by policies and issues could mark the first steps toward supplanting "formal association" with "meaningful social interaction."[50]

Propelled by a commitment to finding out "just how they feel," just what the proposals mean for their lives—specifically, for *their* lives, not for lives that appear superficially to be like theirs—such conversations could work toward reducing the defensiveness in which instrumental, bureaucratic moves often issue. Finding out how they feel does not mean accepting their every utterance as immune to critical discussion, for then tolerance would become an indifferent refusal to debate, to engage with one another in intelligent, democratic dialogue. Rather, finding out how they feel means participating with them in policy-making processes, where it is just as possible for 'them' as it is for 'us' to set the agenda; recognizing that similarities between points of view cannot be assumed, have always to be debated, and that in consequence of a responsibly engaged conversation, all of the participants may feel quite differently. The process requires no disingenuous denial of the specialized knowledge that may inform the (traditionally) 'expert' side; yet it demands a careful exploration, case by case, of the pertinence and the limitations of expertise.

These suggestions are not merely idealistic pie in the sky. Admittedly, successful instances are rare in bureaucratic societies, but there is evidence that they are proliferating, for example, as urban planners manifest a renewed sensitivity to what it means to live in neighborhoods; as environmental policies are differently sensitive to issues specific to each separate region; as distributors of foreign aid try to find out what kind of aid is appropriate, as they resist simply imposing a first world standard, in a projection of how they think *they* would feel. Nor can any solution be touted as the absolute, final one. Even the most complex and costly of democratically agreed solutions may have to be redone, and sooner rather than later, as circumstances evolve beyond what the problem solvers could have foretold. To be ready for such eventualities, it is important to preserve the ambiguity that empathetic knowing, paradoxically, requires.

Notes

I am grateful to Peta Bowden and Richard Schmitt for extensive comments on an earlier version of this paper, and to members of the audience at the conferences and meetings where I have presented all or part of it for discussion.

1. Kathy Ferguson, *The Feminist Case against Bureaucracy* (Philadelphia: Temple University Press, 1984), 13–14.

2. Ibid., 9, 31.

3. Ferguson notes similarities with Jacques Ellul's technical civilization,

characterized by "deference to and dependence upon a very limited notion of rationality . . . , artificiality . . . , automatism . . . , and universalism" (ibid., 34).

4. Michel Foucault, *Discipline and Punish: The Birth of the Prison*, trans. Alan Sheridan (New York: Vintage Books, 1979), 191. Quoted in Ferguson, *The Feminist Case*, 137.

5. Wittgenstein writes: "Grammar tells us what kind of object anything is. (Theology as grammar)." Ludwig Wittgenstein, *Philosophical Investigations*, trans. G.E.M. Anscombe (Oxford: Basil Blackwell, 1951), #373.

6. See, for example, Jean Baker Miller, *Toward a New Psychology of Women* (Boston: Beacon Press, 1976). The phrase 'affiliative qualities' is Marcia Westkott's, in "Female Rationality and the Idealized Self," *American Journal of Psychoanalysis* 49:3 (1989):239–250, 239. Yet Westkott has serious reservations about the emancipatory potential of an ideally empathetic female self, whose required self-abnegation may issue only in a perpetual submissiveness.

7. My point is not to posit a radical distinction between ethical theories that make justice central and those that privilege care, but to highlight a difference between them where issues of gender figure prominently. See Claudia Card, "Gender and Moral Luck," *Identity, Character, and Morality*, ed. Owen Flanagan and Amelie Rorty (Cambridge, Mass.: M.I.T. Press, 1990).

8. Ferguson, *The Feminist Case*, 76, refers to the control strategies of managerial discourse, where "objective" standards for performance evaluation "take the basic human abilities to take the perspective of the other, to empathize, to treat others with dignity and respect, and break them down into minute subcategories, thereby transforming them into nonhuman categories."

9. Owen Flanagan and Kathryn Jackson, "Justice, Care, and Gender: The Kohlberg-Gilligan Debate Revisited," *Ethics* 97 (April 1987):622–637, 623.

10. For a discussion of responsible epistemic practice, see my *Epistemic Responsibility* (Hanover, N.H.: University Press of New England, 1987); and, for the present context, my "Persons, and Others," in *Power, Gender, Values*, ed. Judith Genova (Edmonton: Academic Printing and Publishing, 1987).

11. See chapter 3 of my *What Can She Know? Feminist Theory and the Construction of Knowledge* (Ithaca, N.Y.: Cornell University Press, 1991). Baier observes: "A person, perhaps, is best seen as one who was long enough dependent upon other persons to acquire the essential arts of personhood. Persons essentially are *second* persons." Annette Baier, "Cartesian Persons," in Baier, *Postures of the Mind: Essays on Mind and Morals* (Minneapolis: University of Minnesota Press, 1985), 84. Emphasis added.

12. Marilyn Frye, *The Politics of Reality* (Trumansburg, N.Y.: Crossing Press, 1983), 80.

13. See especially Nancy Chodorow, *The Reproduction of Mothering: Psy-*

choanalysis and the Sociology of Gender (Berkeley: University of California Press, 1978).

14. Ferguson, *The Feminist Case,* 159.

15. Westkott, "Female Rationality," 24. Emphasis added.

16. For arguments against such naturalistic assumptions, even about childbirth, see Virginia Held, "Birth and Death," in *Feminism and Political Theory,* ed. Cass R. Sunstein (Chicago: University of Chicago Press, 1990); Emily Martin, *The Woman in the Body: A Cultural Analysis of Reproduction* (Boston: Beacon Press, 1987).

17. Nel Noddings observes that her book *Caring* has drawn the charge of parochialism. Yet her goal is to promote a kind of moral education that would promote "ever-widening circles of caring." Nel Noddings, "The Alleged Parochialism of Caring," *American Philosophical Association Feminism and Philosophy Newsletter* 90:2 (Winter 1991) 96–99, 97.

18. Quoted in Alfred Margulies, *The Empathic Imagination* (New York: W. W. Norton and Co., 1989), xi.

19. Ibid., 3, 4.

20. David M. Berger, *Clinical Empathy* (Northvale, N.J. : Aronson, 1987), 6.

21. See, for example, Ruth Ginzberg, "Uncovering Gynocentric Science," *Hypatia: A Journal of Feminist Philosophy* 2:3 (Fall 1987):89–105; Jane Roland Martin, *Reclaiming a Conversation: The Ideal of the Educated Woman* (New Haven: Yale University Press, 1985), chap. 5, "Beecher's Homemakers"; Londa Schiebinger, *The Mind Has No Sex? Women in the Origins of Modern Science* (Cambridge, Mass.: Harvard University Press, 1989), chap. 4, "Women's Traditions"; Linda Alcoff and Vrinda Dalmiya, "Are 'Old Wives' Tales' Justified?," in *Feminist Epistemologies,* ed. Linda Alcoff and Libby Potter (New York: Routledge, 1993); chap. 6, "Credibility: A Double Standard," of my *What Can She Know?*

22. Westkott, "Female Rationality," 243.

23. Margulies, *The Empathic Imagination,* 18.

24. These symmetries prevail even though therapy itself is often represented as a 'feminized' branch of medicine and even though there are many female therapists, some of whom practice according to a traditional 'male' model.

25. Ferguson, *The Feminist Case,* 142, 144.

26. See in this connection chapter 6, "Credibility: A Double Standard," in my *What Can She Know?* See also Barbara Ehrenreich and Deirdre English, *For Her Own Good: 150 Years of the Experts' Advice to Women* (New York: Doubleday, 1978).

27. Ferguson, *The Feminist Case,* 22, 56.

28. Susan Hekman, *Gender and Knowledge: Elements of a Postmodern Feminism* (Boston: Northeastern University Press, 1990), 4.

29. By 'pre-interpretive' I mean closed to the possibilities that interpreta-

tion offers, devoted to 'just the facts,' convinced that positivist methods alone will do.

30. See for example, Albert O. Hirschman, "The Search for Paradigms as a Hindrance to Understanding," in *Interpretive Social Science*, ed. Paul Rabinow and William Sullivan (Berkeley: University of California Press, 1987).

31. Paul Rabinow and William Sullivan, "The Interpretive Turn: A Second Look," in *Interpretive Social Science*, ed. Rabinow and Sullivan, 7.

32. For an instructive discussion of interpretation, see Joseph Rouse, *Knowledge and Power: Toward a Political Philosophy of Science* (Ithaca, N.Y.: Cornell University Press, 1987), chap. 3; and see Kathy Ferguson, "Interpretation and Genealogy in Feminism," *Signs: Journal of Women in Culture and Society* 16:2 (Winter 1991):322–339, for a debate that pertains to the present context.

33. Michelle Z. Rosaldo, "Moral/Analytic Dilemmas Posed by the Intersection of Feminism and Social Science," in *Interpretive Social Science*, ed. Rabinow and Sullivan, 291, 292.

34. Henrietta Moore, *Feminism and Anthropology* (Minneapolis: University of Minnesota Press, 1988), 25.

35. See, for example, Lynda Birke, *Women, Feminism, and Biology* (Brighton: Harvester Press, 1986); Ruth Hubbard, Mary Sue Henifin, and Barbara Fried, eds., *Biological Woman—The Convenient Myth* (Cambridge, Mass.: Schenkman Publishing Company, 1982); Janet Sayers, *Biological Politics* (London: Tavistock Publications, 1982). See also Thomas Laqueur, *Making Sex: Body and Gender from the Greeks to Freud* (Cambridge, Mass.: Harvard University Press, 1990).

36. Rosaldo, "Moral/Analytic Dilemmas," 293.

37. Thomas Nagel, *The Possibility of Altruism* (Princeton: Princeton University Press, 1970), 15.

38. Nancy J. Holland, *Is Women's Philosophy Possible?* (Savage, Md.: Rowman & Littlefield, 1990), 43.

39. Robert Hogan, "Moral Conduct and Moral Character: A Psychological Perspective," *Psychological Bulletin* 79:4 (April 1973):217–232, 222, emphasis added.

40. Ibid., 223.

41. Moore, *Feminism and Anthropology*, 186.

42. Margulies, *The Empathic Imagination*, 12, 18, 142.

43. Ferguson, *The Feminist Case*, 7. Emphasis added.

44. Simone de Beauvoir, *The Ethics of Ambiguity*, trans. Bernard Frechtman (New York: Citadel Press, 1962), 108. In my reading of this text, I am indebted to Catriona A. Mackenzie, "Embodying Autonomy: Women and Moral Agency" (Ph.D. dissertation, Australian National University, 1991), esp. chaps. 2–3.

45. De Beauvoir, *The Ethics of Ambiguity*, 17.

46. See Hekman, *Gender and Knowledge*, 73–79.

47. Ibid., 67.

48. 'Facticity,' in the writings of Sartre and de Beauvoir, refers to the intransigent facts of embodiment, mortality, finitude: the aspects of human being and of the world that are resistant to the human will. Facticity limits freedom; but without it freedom would be impossible.

49. De Beauvoir, *The Ethics of Ambiguity*, 136. For de Beauvoir, "one of the concrete consequences of existentialist ethics is the rejection of all the previous justifications which might be drawn from the civilization, the age, and the culture; it is the rejection of every principle of authority," 142; "man is man only through situations whose particularity is precisely a universal fact," 144.

50. Ferguson, *The Feminist Case*.

JOAN A. LANG

Is Empathy Always "Nice"?
Empathy, Sympathy, and the Psychoanalytic Situation

During my clinical rotation on pediatrics as a medical student, one of seven women in a class of seventy-five, I "rounded" one day (the process of following an attending physician on his medical rounds on a teaching hospital ward to visit and discuss the cases of patients) with a pediatric surgeon of immense intelligence and enthusiasm, whom I idolized then (and still admire greatly). The group also included several of my male classmates. As we approached the bed of a five-year-old girl, Dr. R. remarked that he hated visiting this patient because she screamed from the first sight of him until the examination ended. Indeed, as soon as she spotted us, she began to shriek. He attempted to teach us, over the sound of her pathetic (but shrill and irritating) cries, about the rare cancer from which she suffered. After a while, I moved to the head of her bed, took her hand, and said, kindly but firmly, "There now, you hush and be a good girl. We're not going to hurt you." To my surprise—and the respectful amazement of my attending and envy of my classmates—she quieted immediately. Gripping my hand, she cooperated with the exam. As we began to leave, the child spoke for the first time, calling after us (me): "I *was* a good girl, wasn't I?" Moved, I returned, squeezed her hands, and replied "Yes! You were a *very* good girl." Then I hurried on to rejoin the rounds. She (and my success with her) stayed in my mind off and on during the busy days of a third-year medical student. Several days later, I found time to return to her ward to visit her. But in the meantime, she had died.

I have processed this incident in a variety of ways over the years. I have come to see it as revealing much about the atmosphere of medical training, of gender roles in a manpower system, and of what values are fostered or neglected in even the best educational institutions. I have pondered the power of the "good girl" injunction that compels so many of us to order our lives and even our deaths to please others. But here I would like to examine the perspectives on empathy we can glean from it, particularly on what in this incident we would consider to illustrate empathy, and what not—and why or why not.

From there, I will explore the meaning of empathy in the special context of the psychoanalytic situation, particularly as it has been elaborated within the body of psychoanalytic theory and practice known as the psychology of the self. Although I will allude to some of the implications for understanding empathy in a larger context of experience, I will draw mainly on the powerful and significant role of empathy in therapeutic settings. It allows patient and analyst to explore together the inner world of complex, conscious, and unconscious mental life—for one person to understand the subjective reality of another. My specific thesis is that empathy is best characterized as a way of understanding the inner experience of others, and that the insight thus gained can be put to many uses, only some of which may be therapeutic or "nice."

Empathy?—First Take

Naturally, I first believed myself to have demonstrated an impressive natural talent for empathy. I had read the little girl's distress—who could miss it?! But further, and unlike my insensitive male medical colleagues (even my revered attending physician), I had sensed her fear and what would quiet it: personal attention, a comforting hand. And I had supplied these things. This all happened long before I had become in any way enlightened as a feminist thinker. (After all, I had suffered no gender discrimination; therefore it did not exist. It is embarrassing to recall how much my naïveté, self-interest, privilege, and the need to fit in enabled me to deny and overlook.) So I don't think I asked myself then, or for a long time afterwards, whether my apparent empathic sensitivity might reflect a gender-based role more than a personal gift. What I mostly felt, when I would remember the incident from time to time over the next few years, included sadness at her death, some regret or even guilt that I had not made time to return to see her before she died, but mostly—consciously—pride that my natural empathy had enabled me to make a so-impressive showing, and showing up of my rivals, before our esteemed leader.

Second Take

At some point in my later personal psychoanalysis, I found myself viewing the story from a very different angle—one, indeed, that turned triumph into shame. I realized that my "sensitivity" had been put to the use of self-aggrandizement, and that the dying child was relegated to the role of a bit player in my drama of impressing my mentor and defeating my rivals. I completely revised my judgment on my actions, which in this new light seemed the very opposite of empathic. Indeed, some years later, in a paper titled "Becoming a Better Therapist," I used this story to illustrate "pseudo-empathy"—as an object lesson, albeit from a brief experience rather than a longer and more intimate psychotherapeutic encounter, on what empathy is not: neither sympathy nor a kind of superficial rapport organized around self rather than other, used to exploit the other for the agendas and needs of oneself.[1]

Empathy: Take Three

But what does it mean to assess my past self in this encounter as "being empathic" or not? Or more precisely, as exhibiting, or failing to exhibit, accurate empathy? On reevaluation, I have come to think that I *was* in fact empathic—but not very "nice." I would now say that my perceptions were empathic: I did accurately perceive her feeling state and her needs. So my actions, or interventions, with the little girl were empathically informed. Were they sympathetic? In outcome, they were probably so experienced *by her*—she felt better during this exam than others, perhaps gained some feeling of self-esteem and approval from "being good," had her hand held in a comforting way. But what of *my* relationship to the empathically gained data? In what way must we take account of my motivations, which were more selfish than generous (though including genuine sympathy, too; these things are always complex), more attuned to my own agendas than to her needs? What of my actions, which exploited her needs for comfort and approval in the service of shutting her up as much as soothing her? Can we refer to a manipulative use of another person as "empathic," and, if so, must that person experience the transaction as "nice"?

In asking such questions of this seemingly simple exchange, we begin to approach various complex distinctions: the point of view of the person exercising empathy versus that of the recipient of the resulting action; motivations or intentions of the empathizer versus actual outcomes; conscious versus unconscious intentions; and the meaning(s) that the experience has for both participants, which may be very different. From the perspective of the empathizer, the fundamental activity is mental: perceiving and understanding the inner feelings of another. But when we consider empathy from the point of view of the person receiving it, we are inclined to look at actions and the quality of subjectively experienced outcomes. Thus it is when we speak of "being empathic" that confusion arises, because so often we wish to imply "being sympathetic" or "nice" (that is, caring, good, benevolent, therapeutic) rather than simply being accurately attuned.

I now believe that this sad and telling story illustrates a distinction central to the definition of empathy as Heinz Kohut conceptualizes it in his theory of the psychology of the self.[2] Empathy as a mental activity stands at the very center of self psychology—indeed, for Kohut empathy is *the* definer of the field of psychoanalysis as a scientific discipline.[3] But "empathy" and "sympathy" are to be sharply distinguished. Empathy is defined as a mode of perception or observation, usually including (but not limited to) listening; it is a mode of data gathering. As such, it is, or should be, value-neutral. In fact, to be accurate, empathic immersion (also termed "vicarious introspection" by Kohut) *must* be neutral if it is to succeed in its goal of perceiving the subjective experience of the other without imposing external values upon the data being apprehended. Kohut further insisted that accurate attunement—and the data gathered by empathic immersion—need not lead to sympathy, that it could be put to hostile as well as benign uses. He liked to cite the example of the Nazis' use of diabolically empathic devices (such as attaching howling sirens to their dive bombers, knowing well how the sounds would add to the terror) to illustrate this point.[4]

What *is* the relation between empathy and sympathy? People often treat them as synonyms, which is, I would argue, a serious source of confusion. In psychoanalytic circles, one of the most devastating criticisms leveled at self psychology is that its emphasis on the centrality of empathy encourages "cure through sympathy" or "just being nice to your patients." This is considered a severe attack because it seems to self psychologists to miss the whole point, outlined above, of what empathy is. Moreover, it is considered a severe attack because, if true, such a charge would exclude this form of treatment from being taken seriously as psychoanalysis, as depth psychology, or as "scientific medicine."[5] To explore these questions more thoroughly, I will now leave my starting place, the story presented, to launch further considerations of empathy by reviewing it as a central construct within self psychology.

Heinz Kohut, Empathy, and Self Psychology: A Brief History

A brief review of self psychology will help to orient those readers for whom it is not a familiar theoretical framework. It is important to appreciate that the approach now known as self psychology (or the psychology of the self) began not as a challenge to mainstream psychoanalytic thinking but as a development from within it. Heinz Kohut was trained in medicine at the University of Vienna, in neurology and psychiatry at the University of Chicago, and in the classical tradition of Freudian psychoanalysis at the Chicago Institute for Psychoanalysis, where he continued to work as faculty and training analyst. In 1959 he published "Introspection, Empathy, and Psychoanalysis: An Examination of the Relationship Between Mode of Observation and Theory" in the *Journal of the American Psychoanalytic Association*;[6] he was to look back on this paper as setting forth the kernel of his later work. But it was in the years between 1966, when he wrote the paper "Forms and Transformations of Narcissism," which was to become the nucleus of his first book, *The Analysis of the Self* (1971), and his death in 1981 that he became known as the originator of the psychology of the self.[7] He initially presented his shift in theoretical conceptualizations and technical recommendations as a relatively discrete (and discreet?) contribution to classical psychoanalytic theory, concerned with a particular subgroup of patients who were especially narcissistically vulnerable—that is, fragile and disturbed in their fundamental sense of self. Quickly, however, Kohut and his students and co-workers extended the reach of his formulations, until many saw self psychology as a "supraordinate" theoretical framework that not only complemented but superseded much of classical theory.

I focus here only on Kohut's views on empathy. Two observations are most relevant to my discussion. First, Kohut emphasized empathy as *the* definitively psychoanalytic mode of data gathering. He repeatedly stressed his conviction that only immersion within the patient's subjective experience, what he called "vicarious introspection," could provide the information about complex mental states that is the purview of psychoanalysis. Second, according to Kohut's account, his theoretical elaboration emerged from his ongoing experiences of clinical practice. He wrote of patients who insisted that he was "not listening" and whose persistent complaints in the face of his seemingly correct (in classical theoretical terms) interpretations demonstrated their need for different ways of understanding and interpreting their experience. It is not too extreme to state that self psychology as a theory grew out of Kohut's commitment to privileging empathically gained knowledge over the knowledge he had acquired through his training. By attempting to keep as closely attuned as possible to his patients' unfolding experiences, including their transference configurations,[8] without imposing premature, theory-based (what he called "experience-distant") interpretations onto them, Kohut arrived at new perspectives on their material. In turn, as he used these newly available perspectives, and made interpretations based on them—always attempting to maintain a rigorously empathic stance toward his patients' experience (versus his own intentions or attitudes) as he interpreted—he saw new transference configurations unfold. Previously unavailable feelings and memories became available to him for analysis and interpretation.

Two books, *The Restoration of the Self* (1977)[9] and *How Does Analysis Cure?* (posthumously published in 1984),[10] and numerous papers elaborated a theory of mental health, psychological development and psychopathology, and psychoanalytic treatment. In all of these, empathy recurs as a central motif. Just how central it was to Kohut may be seen by his return to considerations of empathy in both his final public address, "Reflections on Empathy," delivered three days before his death,[11] and in his last paper, "Introspection, Empathy, and the Semi-Circle of Mental Health," published posthumously in 1982.[12]

In these works, Kohut made several important distinctions about empathy. First, he distinguished the "epistemological context," or empathy defined in relationship to knowledge—its acquisition and its use in formulating theories: "In this context, as should go without saying, empathy is a value-neutral mode of observation; a mode of observation attuned to the inner life of man, just as extrospection is a mode of observation attuned to the external world."[13] Second, he addressed (as he had not done in his 1959 essay) empathy in an "empirical context, as a mental *activity*, whether employed in every day life, or in scientific pursuits." In approaching empathy in this context, which struck Kohut as a "more complex but still manageable undertaking," he believed that "we must differentiate between two levels: (1) empathy as an information-gathering activity, and (2) empathy as a powerful emotional bond between people." Most significantly, he stressed that "as an information-collecting, data-gathering activity, empathy, as I have stressed many times since 1971, can be right or wrong, in the service of compassion or hostility, pursued slowly and ploddingly or 'intuitively,' that is, at great speed. In this sense empathy is never by itself supportive or therapeutic. It is, however, a necessary precondition to being successfully supportive and therapeutic."[14]

Kohut is saying here that empathy is a necessary but not a sufficient condition for therapeutic responses. Correct interventions must be guided by accurate empathy, which *informs* but does not guarantee them. In fact, hostile or self-serving actions can be informed by accurate empathy—and will be the more devastating when they are so informed (we always know how best to hurt, as well as help, the one we love).

Kohut was more ambivalent about empathy as a powerful emotional bond between people:

> I wish that I could stop my discussion of empathy as a concrete force in human life at this point without having to make one further step, which appears to contradict everything I have said so far, and which exposes me to the suspicion of abandoning scientific sobriety and of entering the land of mysticism or of sentimentality. I assure you that I would like to avoid making this step and that it is not the absence of scientific rigor but submission to it that forces me to tell you that even though everything I have said up to now remains fully valid so long as we evaluate empathy as an instrument of observation and as an informer of . . . action . . . I must now, *unfortunately*, add that empathy per se, the mere presence of empathy, has also a beneficial, in a broad sense, a therapeutic effect—both in the clinical setting and in human life, in general."[15]

Why "unfortunately"? Why was Kohut so reluctant to acknowledge that empathy itself has a beneficial effect? Surely common sense would tell us this. Most people will tolerate (and might even provoke) hostile attention from someone who recognizes and, albeit perversely, comprehends their essential significance far better than they will the chilling effects of indifference and unconnectedness. And, indeed, questions about the curative effect of the empathic bond were among the most frequent that Kohut, often impatiently, received from his readers, students, and critics. In his last public appearance, he ruefully reflected on how long it had taken him to admit that anything that so many people kept on asking must be a "real" question, requiring genuine attention and reformulation.[16] A full discussion of the background to his reluctance would take us far afield, but I believe some of the most relevant factors include:

1. The longstanding anxiety of psychoanalysts since Freud that our discipline may not be respected unless it can lay claim to full status as a science. This leads to a tendency to reject any association with "irrational" elements (as empathy is often considered to be) which might, as Kohut mused, "expose [one] to the suspicion of abandoning scientific sobriety";
2. The concern of Kohut and his colleagues that self psychology not be extruded from psychoanalysis as being "not really analysis";
3. A long history within psychoanalysis of holding in disrepute an approach termed "the corrective emotional experience"; and
4. A serious concern that the fundamental and necessary neutrality of the analyst would be abandoned if the existence of a "really"

important (as versus fantasized and only transferentially important) bond between patient and analyst were to be recognized.

Isn't "Being Empathic" Really "Being Nice"?

If I do not share these sources of ambivalence toward the inherently desirable impact of empathy on human relationships, what then is the significance of insisting (as I do) on maintaining the firm distinction between empathy and sympathy, or "being nice"? Is such a distinction a semantic quibble? A technicality useful only at the abstract level of epistemology to which Kohut referred? It is neither. I would argue for retaining both a claim to an innate human preference, yearning, and need for empathy, and also that empathy is in itself value-neutral. Potentially it can be motivated by, and used in the service of, hostility or compassion, self-serving exploitativeness or therapeutic benevolence. Consider a few of the clinically and socially common situations which a distinction between empathy and sympathy helps us to explain:

- Charming sociopaths, successful con men, certain used car salespersons
- "Good" (that is, diabolically effective) prosecuting attorneys
- "Guilt-inducers" (how else do they know exactly which buttons to push?)
- Abusive and destructive relationships in which the abusee infuriatingly reports, "I *know* (s)he's bad for me, but when things are good, they're *SO* good!"[17]

Furthermore, careful specification of what empathy is and what it is not will protect us from overgeneralizing the concept into meaninglessness. It is all too easy to equate empathy, or "the empathic physician," with all of the qualities of "good" (that is, responsible, compassionate, caring) therapeutic conduct. For example, a study that attempted to assess the degree to which observers evaluated empathy as an independent quality of a therapeutic interview suggested that there seemed to be no difference between the judges' global ratings of "good" or "effective" interventions and their assessments of the interviewers' empathy—leading the authors to question whether we really know what we mean by the term "empathy," let alone how to measure it.[18] Although it is hard to overstate the importance of empathy, it is easy to sentimentalize it. Kohut warned, "we must beware of mythologizing empathy, this irreplaceable but by no means infallible depth-psychological tool. Empathy is not God's gift bestowed only on an elect few."[19]

"Fiendish Empathy": Why Do We Hate the Concept?

I have been surprised to find in many audiences a persistent and even impassioned rejection of the very idea that there can be "bad" empathy. In response to examples cited, objectors will say that one demonstrates an imperfect empathy, another perhaps an abuse of empathy—but that it is unacceptable to consider that someone who is "fiendish," sadistic, or even merely exploitative is empathic. Is it possible that empathy has been idealized and overvalued?[20]

Let us consider in some detail a clinical example that centrally involves what I would consider to be empathy put to destructive uses. I have for some years been devoting special study to what I have called the "Addictive Bad Object." This is the situation familiar to anyone who has grieved and worried over repetitively entering into relationships with "bad objects"—that is, unsuitable others with whom the hapless victim falls hopelessly in love despite every prompting of experience, better judgment, and the pleas of friends. For example, a smart, otherwise savvy, and articulate professional woman, whom I will call Karen, put it thus about her manipulative, substance-abusing, unfaithful lover: "Of course, I *know* she's bad for me, but it's only when I'm with her that I feel truly myself, fully alive." Struggling to understand the attraction (which was demonstrated over time and across other relationships to be as compelling, driven, self-destructive, yet irresistible as any addiction), I asked my patient to try to convey to me the source and the quality of the compelling attraction. It was complicated, of course, but what emerged was a pattern visible in other relationships, with roots in her earliest childhood relationships, with resulting conscious and unconscious beliefs, fears, wishes, and defenses, all of which we ultimately explored in the transference relationship with me. The pattern we discovered has turned out to be a meaningful formulation for other patients as well. Again and again, the lover had a very special way of looking deeply into my patient's eyes, of listening intently to her, of laughing at her jokes, of making her feel seen and heard for who she was—in sum, of affirming my patient, of giving her what self psychology terms "mirroring." The reader may well be wondering how this description differs from any infatuation or falling in love, and indeed it does not—except for the crucial particular that my patient could not rely on the continued presence of this valued and enlivening quality of relatedness. Much of her time and energy came to be centered on seeking to "read between the lines," to divine the subtle clues that might reveal the unwritten rules by which the needed and yearned-for mirroring was dispensed or withheld. The only reliable pattern Karen ever recognized was that her lover sensed unerringly any moment at which she had "had about enough," and turned up the wattage long enough to draw her in again.

My clinical work with patients is concerned with analyzing the patient's contribution to this complex relational choreography, and I recognize the pitfalls in attempting to infer at a distance the psychology of the patient's "other." (Unfortunately, as is true of batterers, rapists, and even "Don Juans," it is rare to see the abuser rather than the abusee in the analyst's office, a serious limitation on gathering data and on generating hypotheses.) Nonetheless, the patterns I have observed in a number of patients like Karen have led me to a hypothesis: that persons, like Karen's lover, who present as such charismatic but exploitative "addictive bad objects" possess a capacity for an unusually accurate and finely tuned empathy. They also demonstrate a kind of inner radar for detecting and zeroing in on those potential victims whose emotional history and neediness render them "mirror-hungry" and thus vulnerable to this cruelly tantalizing play on their hopes of having their needs finally met.[21] To me, the "talent" of such persons is an example of "fiendish empathy."

Why would we want to rename this hypothesized talent, to call it something other than empathy? Linguistic meanings are conventions, certainly, and it is logically acceptable to define empathy as "good," inventing other terms for situations in which some kind of attunement is put to malign use. But what is the rationale, what is gained, by doing so? More interestingly, can any rational argument explain the intensity with which many reject the definition suggested here? I am inclined to speculate that there is an inner resistance in all of us that grows from the same soil as the vulnerability of women like the patient I just described. We *all* hunger, forever, for "good" empathy, needing and yearning to be truly understood—so deeply that to consider an empathy that could betray us is repugnant. Like the myth of "maternal instinct," a belief in an inherently benign empathy would promise some protection against this horrifying potential source of violation.

The Empathic Therapist: Considerations of Ethics and Responsibility

If the definitions and the hypotheses I am advancing are correct, then a heavy responsibility rests on therapists who would enhance their empathic reach. If empathy can yield intimate and potentially potent information about others, and if all or many patients are vulnerable to awakened hopes and needs that mobilize deeply rooted, yet conflicted and fragile, parts of themselves, then it would clearly be better all around if empathic knowledge guaranteed sympathetic responses. The therapeutic relationship becomes much scarier if we realize that there is no such built-in guarantee. One is reminded, both inevitably and appropriately, of the erotic longings that likewise can be mobilized in the intimacy and high wattage of the therapeutic dyad. Abuses can happen, and, sadly, they do. Nor can we write off all such incidents as being the property of a few "bad apples": sometimes the offenders have been, save for the lapse, respected and talented therapists of good training and goodwill. Responsible professionals must recognize that virtue and kind intentions confer no immunity. Vigilance, training, ongoing self-analysis, consultation, and careful attention to the countertransference are all necessary to ensure the safety and trustworthiness of our invitations to patients to reveal their vulnerable, undefended selves. It is part of my argument here that we improve the odds of recognizing the dangers if we are not misled by a definition of empathy that would exclude its potential for harm as well as for benefit.

Empathy with What?

One of the most central discoveries and emphases of psychoanalysis is that of the dynamic unconscious—that is to say, the existence in all of us of an active and powerful set of meanings, feelings, conflicts, wishes, needs, desires, defenses, and motivations that are not part of our consciously experienced thought. Indeed, it may be inaccurate to speak of anyone as having a *self* in some singular, wholly cohesive sense. Instead we all possess to a greater or lesser degree, more so at some times and places than others, a multiplicity of potential "selves"—some of them disavowed by, and repugnant to, the conscious and public persona we prefer to present to the world. It is the special job of psychoanalysis to unearth these hidden and repudiated parts of the patient's (and, inevitably, of the analyst's) self so that they become available for new understanding, interpretation, reintegration, and healing (in Kohut's word, "restoration"). It is the special difficulty of psychoanalysis that such material in the unconscious has been repressed for what seemed at the time to be very compelling reasons, and its rediscovery is vigorously opposed by resistances and defenses—again, even when the conscious self is motivated to participate in the analysis. Thus arises a question put to self psychology by many critics (perhaps most notably by Otto Kernberg): "With what does the analyst empathize?"[22] When accurate empathic attunement alerts the analyst to something her patient wishes to avoid, the analytic work of confrontation may feel very *unnice*—unsympathetic, unfeeling, critical, even hostile and threatening to the patient.

A clinical example: Don, a successful lawyer in his fourth year of analysis with me, reports with some agitation an encounter with a senior partner in his law firm the day before. The older man had sent a memo to Don telling him that some important citations had not been included in a document Don had prepared, and saying that this oversight must be corrected as soon as possible. Don was infuriated, and launched into a detailed and scathing account of the other's deficiencies. It was easy to identify with his anger, but I was struck by the degree to which Don seemed "unmanned" by the experience. I asked him to tell me in more detail about the way he had felt at the moment he read the memo. He became impatient with me: "I'm telling you! I felt furious! I still do. I don't see why I should even need to explain it— *anybody* would hate being treated like that!" "Treated like what?" I asked him. His anger at me increased; he began to reexperience the same configuration of feelings and perceptions in the relationship with me. It was only over the course of this session and the next that we were eventually able to reach his feelings of shame and humiliation. These feelings evoked a hated, disavowed, and strongly defended-against self experience of being a helpless and somehow inferior, defective little boy, being teased and shamed by a sadistic and powerful bully. His anger, though real, represented a reactive and preferred "angry man" self experience. Operating on the principle that "the best defense is a good offense," he mobilized this "angry man" and hoped that my "empathy" with this version of his reported experience would reinforce the defense, avoiding the seemingly intolerable feelings associated with the hidden, and seemingly unfixable, "defective self."

Some of the problems connected with this issue of discrepancies between patients' conscious and unconscious needs can be addressed through adjustments in the timing and phrasing of interpretations. But not all. The analyst must be prepared for periods, sometimes lasting much longer than the rather routine example just described, when the patient accuses her or him of being cruel, unfeeling, unempathic, and not at all nice. To further complicate matters, it is always possible that the complaining, "resisting" patient will turn out to be right, and the analyst's quest for empathic attunement with warded-off contents of the self may prove to have been misguided. Such instances—which

Kohut believed to be far more common than the traditional psychoanalytic stance allowed for—are occasions of rupture in the empathic milieu, of (in self psychological terminology) a break in the selfobject bond that had existed in the transference. In effect, the analyst has iatrogenically reinflicted a failure of empathy on the patient. When this occurs, self psychology stresses that the central focus of the analytic work must be on acknowledging and seeking to reconstruct what happened in the patient's experience, and then analyzing how this current empathic failure seemed to repeat past traumas. Again, the ethical as well as technical responsibility of the analyst is weighty.

Ralph Greenson, a noted classical psychoanalyst, once observed, "There seems to be a tendency among analysts either to take empathy for granted or to underestimate it."[23] I would amplify his observation to include the tendency to overestimate empathy, or at least to overidealize it. Analysts have always known that the capacity for empathy is crucial to our therapeutic endeavor; Heinz Kohut and the psychology of the self have greatly enhanced our appreciation of its centrality. As Kohut warned, however, we must beware the temptation to "mythologize" empathy. "Being empathic" does not guarantee infallibility. Indeed, it does not even guarantee being "nice."

Notes

1. J. A. Lang, "Reflections on Becoming a Better Therapist over the Years," paper presented at The Cutting Edge Conference, University of California at San Diego, April 1991; available on audiotape from the University of California at San Diego.

2. H. Kohut, "Introspection, Empathy, and Psychoanalysis: An Examination of the Relationship between Mode of Observation and Theory," *Journal of the American Psychoanalytic Association* 7 (1959):459–483 (reprinted in *The Search for the Self: Selected Writings of Heinz Kohut, 1950–1978*, vol. 1, edited and with an introduction by Paul H. Ornstein [New York: International Universities Press, 1978], 295–232); H. Kohut, "Forms and Transformations of Narcissism," *Journal of the American Psychoanalytic Association* 14 (1966):243–272 (also reprinted in *The Search for the Self*, 427–460); H. Kohut, *The Analysis of the Self* (New York: International Universities Press, 1971); H. Kohut, *The Restoration of the Self* (New York: International Universities Press, 1977); H. Kohut, "Two Letters" and "Reflections on Advances in Self-Psychology," in *Advances in Self-Psychology*, ed. A. Goldberg (New York: International Universities Press, 1980); H. Kohut, "Reflections on Empathy," presented at the Berkeley Conference on the *Psychology of the Self*, videotape, Continuing Education Seminars, Los Angeles, Calif., 1981; H. Kohut, *How Does Analysis Cure?* ed. A. Goldberg and P. Stepansky (Chi-

cago: University of Chicago Press, 1984); H. Kohut and E. Wolf, "The Disorders of the Self and Their Treatment: An Outline," *International Journal of Psychoanalysis* 59 (1978):412–425.

3. In a letter to a colleague in September 1978, Kohut wrote: "I have given a good deal of thought to the role and position of empathy in our field—indeed I consider my views here to constitute the basis for the whole of my work, a conclusion that is not idiosyncratic but was also reached by others who studied and evaluated my contributions to depth psychology . . . (the collection [of my selected writings] bears the title *The Search for the Self* [1978]; originally, however it had been my intention to call it *Scientific Empathy and Empathic Science,* a choice which again tells you how crucial I consider my position on empathy to be)." H. Kohut, "Two Letters" (1980).

4. Kohut, "Two Letters" and "Reflections on Advances in Self-Psychology."

5. S. Harding, *Whose Science? Whose Knowledge?* (Ithaca, N.Y.: Cornell University Press, 1991); Evelyn Fox Keller, *Reflections on Gender and Science* (New Haven: Yale University Press, 1985); G. Reed, "The Antithetical Meaning of the Term 'Empathy' in Psychoanalytic Discourse," *Empathy I,* ed. J. Lichtenberg, M. Bornstein, and D. Silver (Hillsdale, N.J.: Analytic Press, 1984), 7–36. The issue of eligibility for the prestige and status of scientific respectability, a significant underpinning to much of the debate within psychiatry over terminology and methods, is beyond the scope of this essay.

6. Kohut, "Introspection, Empathy, and Psychoanalysis."

7. Kohut, *The Analysis of the Self.*

8. Transference in psychoanalytic theory refers to the re-experiencing in the context of a current relationship—in an analysis, particularly in the relationship to the analyst—of important (often unconscious) aspects of old relationships. Transference is ubiquitous and not always pathological. In the analytic setting, crucial therapeutic leverage is derived from the revealing and emotionally convincing quality of transference configurations which can be seen and understood. Classical analytic theory focuses on those configurations which reenact dramas of love and hate, usually originating in the oedipal, or sometimes the preoedipal stage of psychosexual development. One of Kohut's major contributions, acknowledged even by most of his critics, was to demonstrate that analyzable transference configurations (called "selfobject" transferences) could emerge around conflicted or unmet needs for self-cohesion, affirmation (mirroring), and other issues related to early self-development.

9. Kohut, *The Restoration of the Self.*

10. Kohut, *How Does Analysis Cure?.*

11. Kohut, "Reflections on Empathy."

12. Kohut, "Introspection, Empathy, and the Semi-Circle of Mental Health," *International Journal of Psycho-Analysis,* 63 (1982):395–408.

13. Kohut, *How Does Analysis Cure?* 84.

14. Ibid., 85.

15. Ibid. Emphasis added.

16. Note that an "empathic stance" is here being adopted by Kohut toward his questioners, parallel to that which his theory directs therapists to adopt toward patients. This extension of the role of empathy in data gathering has been further explicated by Paul Ornstein in an interesting set of recommendations on how to listen to (or read) and discuss the papers or case reports of colleagues. See P. Ornstein, "How to 'Enter' a Psychoanalytic Process Conducted by Another Analyst: A Self Psychology View," *Psychoanalytic Inquiry* 10:4 (1990):478–497.

17. J. A. Lang, "The Passionate Self: One + One," paper presented at a conference entitled "Passionate Attachments," University of California at Los Angeles Extension, October 20, 1985 (audiotape from Continuing Education Seminars, Los Angeles, Calif.).

18. H. J. Bachrach, "Empathy: We Know What We Mean, But What Do We Measure?" *Archives of General Psychiatry* 3 (1976):35–38.

19. Kohut, *How Does Analysis Cure?* 83.

20. In a kind of reverse parallel to the devaluing by sentimentalizing of "sympathy" detailed in this volume by Ellen More, there appears to me to be an overvaluing by idealizing of "empathy."

21. Kohut and Wolf, "The Disorders of the Self and Their Treatment: An Outline."

22. O. Kernberg, "Notes on Empathy," *Bulletin of the Association of Psychoanalytic Medicine* 18 (1979):75–80.

23. R. R. Greenson, "Empathy and Its Vicissitudes," *Explorations in Psychoanalysis* (1960; New York: International Universities Press, 1978), 147–161.

JANET L. SURREY AND STEPHEN J. BERGMAN
(SAMUEL SHEM)

Gender Differences in Relational Development

Implications for Empathy in the Doctor-Patient Relationship

For the past decade, building on Jean Baker Miller's book *Toward a New Psychology of Women* (1976), the Stone Center at Wellesley College has been formulating a relational perspective on women's psychological development.[1] This self-in-relation model encompasses a sense of "self," and also a sense of the "other" and a sense of the relationship, stressing what Stone Center theorists call "self-with-other" experiences.[2] According to this model, the primary motivation for human beings is not sex, aggression, or narcissism but, rather, the primary desire for connection. Healthy connection implies an awareness of and care for self, other, and the relationship, and none of these can be sacrificed in the search for mutuality. Healthy growth takes place through and toward connection. Developmental differences between women and men, however, can have significant implications for male-female relationships. These may include differences in empathic attunement, in emphasis on mutuality in relationship, and in orientation to relational processes.[3] Gender differences, we believe, may lead to impasses and disconnections that also negatively affect the power of the healing relationship. The implications of these differences for development of mutuality and empathy in the doctor-patient relationship can be especially profound when the relationship is between the two sexes. We believe that the nature of the doctor-patient relationship often closely resembles the prototypical male-female relationship. For example, the power imbalance in this relationship does not foster relational mutuality. Fundamentally, the "professional expert" or "professional authority" role cultivated as "appropriate" in medicine might even be understood as an extension of *male* development. The study of men's relational development then offers new dimensions for understanding the development of the "physician" in Western medicine. For centuries, the model of the "good doctor" has been, in fact, "the good [white] male doctor."

Women's Psychological Development

Surrey, in her 1985 paper "The Self-in-Relation: A Theory of Women's Development," describes the connections, disconnections, and violations that shape women's experience in this culture, including women's carrying the one-sided responsibility for the care and maintenance of relationships.[4] The notion of the self-in-relation shifts the emphasis from separation to relationship as the basis for self-experience and development. Further, relationship is seen as the basic goal of development, that is, the deepening capacity for relationship and relational competence. Healthy growth in connection implies a deepening capacity for participating in mutually empathic and mutually empowering connections. The self-in-relation model assumes that other aspects of self (for example, creativity, autonomy, assertion) develop within this primary context. That is, other aspects of self-development emerge in the context of relationship, and there is no inherent need to disconnect or to sacrifice relationship for self-development. This formulation implies that we must develop an adequate description of relational development in order to understand women's self-development.

Empathy: Gender Implications for the Doctor-Patient Relationship

Surrey has called empathy a "crucial feature" of a self-in-relation model of women's development. Gender differences in the valuing and learning of mutual empathy have profound implications for the gender differences and impasses in the doctor-patient relationship.[5]

Heinz Kohut and D. W. Winnicott emphasized the importance of empathy in the early development of the self, whether male or female.[6] The interest in connections with others, however, seems to be much more prominent for women at all stages of life. Our research and clinical observation show that most women have a greater affinity for relatedness, emotional closeness, and emotional flexibility than do many men. The capacity for empathy, consistently found in our work to be more developed in women, can be seen as the central organizing concept in women's relational experience. Indeed the Stone Center definition of relationship involves an experience of *mutual* empathy.[7] The ability to be in relationship appears to rest on the development of the capacity for empathy in *both* or *all* persons involved.[8] Winnicott's "good enough mother," capable of providing an empathic facilitating environment for the growing child, does not suddenly appear with the birth of the infant. Much unrecognized learning must have taken place to allow the complex capacities for mothering to emerge in response to the changes of the growing child.[9]

Kohut has emphasized the importance of parental empathy and mirroring in the child's early self-development, but almost no attention has been devoted to the topic of *teaching and learning empathy*. Kohut emphasized the profound importance to the developing child of the experience of empathy from early parental figures, without, however, describing the origins of the capacity for empathy.[10] As a result, many construed it as a highly subjective, intuitive, perhaps innate skill, the stuff of romantic novels and the idealization of women.

Instead, the concept of the relational self relies heavily on a new definition of empathy stressing the growth of this capacity as primary in women's development.[11] Jordan has reexamined the significance of empathy in building healthy connections. She has shown that the ability to experience, comprehend, and respond to the inner state of another person is a highly complex process, relying on a high level of psychological development and learning. Accurate empathy involves a balancing of affective arousal and cognitive structures. It requires an ability to build on the experience of identification with the other person to form a cognitive assimilation of this experience as a basis for response. Such capacities imply highly developed emotional and cognitive operations requiring practice, modeling, and feedback in relationships. Rather than an "earth mother," innate, or "essential" feminine quality, empathy is something learned and practiced in relationship, supported by a cultural "norm." This has important implications for the doctor/patient relationship.

The early mother-daughter relationship can be seen as a model of growth in connection. One of the crucial structural aspects of the mother-daughter relationship that supports the process of learning mutual empathy is the girl's ongoing interest and emotional desire to be connected to her mother. A patient of Dr. Surrey's described her three-year-old daughter's frequent questioning of her: "What are you feeling, Mommy?" The mother would respond thoughtfully and carefully to the question. She was puzzled that she hardly recalled such an interaction with her five-year-old son. This early attentiveness to feeling states and the mother's corresponding ease with and interest in emotional sharing may form the basic sense of "learning to listen," to orient and attune to the other person through feelings. A man described his childhood experience as "learning not to listen, to shut out my mother's voice so that I would not be distracted from pursuing my own interests." For girls, "being present with" psychologically is often experienced as self-enhancing, whereas for boys it may come to be experienced as invasive, engulfing, or threatening.

"Being with" means "being seen" and "feeling seen" by the other and "seeing the other" and sensing the other "feeling seen." This is the experience of mutual empathy. Think, for a second, of how differently men and women, especially doctors, know what this means and actually live it in their daily lives and work.

Usually this open connection is not only allowed but encouraged between mothers and daughters. This may be the origin of the process of "seeing through the eyes of the other." When this process does not work, there can be profound disturbances in the relational development and in the psychological well-being of both daughters and mothers.

The basic elements of the core self in women, the self-in-relation, according to the Stone Center model, can be summarized as:

1. An interest in, and attention to, the other person(s) that forms the base for the emotional connection and the ability to empathize with the other(s).
2. The expectation of a mutual empathic process through which the sharing of experience leads to a heightened development of self and other.
3. The expectation of interaction and relationship as a process of mutual sensitivity and mutual responsibility that provides the stimulus for the growth of empowerment and self-knowledge.

The self develops in the context of relationships, rather than as an isolated or separated autonomous individual. This is a two-way interactional model, in which it becomes as important to understand as to be understood, to empower as well as to be empowered. (How different this is from the classic doctor-patient relationship.) Mutuality and movement in relationship is the optimal context for growth and psychological empowerment. All women in this culture do not necessarily follow this pathway, nor do all follow it in the same way, but in general this relational pathway is more highly encouraged and facilitated for girls than for boys. Women are often disempowered and silenced when relationships do not move toward mutuality. They have felt shamed and devalued when the prevailing culture has viewed the relational way of being as "dependent," "overemotional," or "hysterical." This response often characterizes many women's experience in important interactions with male doctors.

In summary, this new theory of women's psychological development has several implications for the impasses that develop when this style of relationship meets the "male" style of relationship, especially in such an emotionally loaded and role-defined arena as the doctor-patient relationship:

1. The interaction is primed to "misfire" in the arena of mutual empathy: the men and women may be speaking two different languages.
2. The disconnections that result can lead to *power* imbalances: the cultural power of the dominant group (men) will be reinforced by the failure of mutual empathy and mutual empowerment. Further, the power imbalances between the two roles—"doctor" and "patient"—will be similarly reinforced, no matter which gender mix is involved.
3. Because there is no absolutely *essential* difference in ability to learn mutual empathy, there is potential to alter relationships toward ones of more mutual empathy, authenticity, and empowerment.
4. Such alteration takes place not from textbooks or lectures but from the experience of learning with others, from the same processes during which such learning takes place in life, that is, growth through and toward connection, with others who are "in the same boat."

Thus to stay in touch with one's own experience of illness and that of one's classmates and colleagues and loved ones, is the most likely pathway for learning the elements of participating in a healthy doctor-patient relationship.

Men's Psychological Development

Most theories of men's development are about a self, not a self-in-relation. Bergman has applied the Stone Center model to men's psychological development.[12] For men as well as women there is a primary desire for connection, and it is less accurate and useful to think of self than to think of self-in-relation, as a process.[13] As with women, the seeds of misery in men's lives are planted in disconnection from others, in isolation, violation, and dominance, and in relationships that are not mutually empowering. To participate in relationships that are not mutual is a source of sadness and rage which, even in the dominant gender, can lead over a period of time to withdrawal, stagnation, and depression, and, characteristically, insecurity, aggression, and violence.

Although there are biological differences between male and female neonates, the first few years of male development are probably quite similar to female development in terms of open emotional connectedness and mutual responsiveness. At about the age of three, sons and mothers begin to relate to each other in a different way from that of daughters and mothers—there is a shift in the relational context. The feelings and impasses that arise around this disconnection have profound implications for the rest of male relational development and the translation of the dominant male power into the institutions of family and society, including medicine. For the male, there is a disconnection from the relationship with mother. The phenomenon we are describing is *not* "separation/individuation" from the mother or psychoanalytic "rejection" of the mother; rather it is a disconnection from the relationship with mother, from the whole relational way of being and growing.[14] Everything in the culture encourages this disconnection as the prelude to "becoming a man." Not only is this a disconnection from the relationship with the mother, but it becomes a disconnection from the very process of relationship itself, a learning by the young boy about turning away from the process of growth in relationship, about turning away from the whole relational mode. A boy is taught to become an *agent of disconnection*. Thus there is a terrible conflict in "normal" male development: between an experience of deep connection with a woman similar to that which female babies experience, and the powerful forces demanding that a boy become an agent of disconnection. This conflict has profound implications for men's relational lives.[15]

This turning away means that the boy never really learns how to do it, how to be in the process with another person and grow. Unlike girls, whose relational development is grounded in the practice of attending and responding to others' feeling states, boys do not get much practice in the arena of empathy. A basic quality of this violation of the relational process is a declaration of difference. The boy sees that he is and must be different from mother and from girls. "Difference" implies comparison—better than or worse than—and may lead to the idea of one person's having power over another. The boy is taught to become someone special, or feel bad if not. Becoming someone special may be at the expense of being with or nurturing others. Over time, becoming a self-in-spite-of-relationship leaves less opportunity to practice relationship. With a growing sense of competence in the world, there is a parallel sense of incompetence in relationship, which may lead the boy and man to feel "I'm not enough in relationship." In a vicious circle of disengagement and achievement, this "I'm not enough" sense can become an impetus for further individualistic striving. The fantasy is that by achieving, a man will win love. Especially when they are in close relationship, some men seem to be in a hurry to get somewhere else and become something else, as if they need to become something else in order to be valued in the relationship they are fleeing to become something else. But no achievement can win love.

Male Doctors as Agents of Disconnection

If one of the "normal" male resolutions of the conflict at the heart of male development is to become an "agent of disconnection," to achieve as a way of "winning love," then the highest achievers in our culture, such as physicians, may be the ones who are least able to learn and grow in connection, or, more important, to help others to do so.

The educational system that selects those who are able to be doctors is based on comparison and competition. Competition implies assertion, and assertion can imply aggression. The slogan is "compare, don't identify." (It is noteworthy that the slogan in Alcoholics Anonymous, a truly "mutual help" organization, is just the opposite: "Identify, Don't Compare." In many ways AA is the model for what a more mutually empathic doctor-patient relationship would look like.) Medical students, especially men, learn to become agents of disconnection. Achievement in this system usually comes at the expense of others' achievement, power at the expense of others' power, helping oneself at the expense of helping others. The highest achievers are those best at competing. They have been taught to learn in isolation and to grow in isolation, and they have not been rewarded for empowering others, nurturing others, or even for helping others in anything remotely resembling true mutuality. Despite medical educators' attempts—after decades of this learning in disconnection to promote self-achievement—to "teach them empathy" (often, in classes using videotapes, telling them to nod their heads and say "Uh-huh" at the right time)—we have difficulty in breaking the cycle at the heart of men's psychological development, of learning to keep themselves out of the process of relationship as a way of growing. Men—and some women—learn to be a self-in-spite-of-relationship.

If the doctor-patient relationship is, at best, one of mutual connection, male doctors are often going against much of what they have been taught. If violations of the doctor-patient relationship (from blatant sexual abuse to emotional coldness and self-protection) result from a combination of self-out-of-relationship stances and inherent power imbalances, male doctors will have great difficulty with issues of sharing power in the doctor-patient relationship.

Medicine reflects society. Society is patriarchal and hierarchical. The fragmentation and violence in our society are reflected in the fragmentation and violence in medicine. Recent studies in the *Journal of the American Medical Association* have shown that 80 percent of medical students report some kind of abuse by the fourth year of medical school, most of it coming in the clinical years, in the large hierarchical systems of the medical centers. No discussion of male development can leave out an analysis of power differences and the potential for violence.[16]

Male violence is epidemic; women are often the victims. In the breakdown of relationship, violence flourishes. The more efficient an agent of disconnection a person becomes, the greater the potential for violence. Violence is a result of disconnection. Nonviolence is the flowering of mutuality.

What is missing from much theory of male development is a power analysis: men denying they have power over women, and men's reaction to the fact of the widespread sexual abuse of girls, women, and young boys. A primary violation in women's lives is the early realization that men are strong and can hurt, physically and sexually. Little girls pick up the violence in a lack of connection—as subtle as a look in a man's eyes, a sexual objectification. Little boys often notice this fear in little girls. Boys learn about their physical power, to enjoy it and to fear it.

While men are taught that they have power and are supposed to act powerfully, men may sense women's fear of it. Men too are afraid of it, in themselves and in other men. In a patriarchy, men may also be victims. Hierarchy means that there is always someone more successful and more powerful, and men are haunted by failure. The biggest winners are potentially the biggest losers. In a "power-over model," it isn't safe to take an authentic, vulnerable, relational stance. In such systems, relationship can be seen as a threat to power. Although a man may find it easy to use power from a self-centered stance, knocking other people over, it is difficult for a man to learn to use power in relationship. Men can come to think that sensitivity to the welfare of others drains power and is hazardous. This fear has grave implications for the doctor-patient relationship in general and gender differences within that context.

Male Relational Dread

We argue that the conflict in "normal" male development—between a positive experience of growth in connection and the cultural imperative to disconnect from relationship to be a man—is a basis for male "relational dread." Male relational dread is a prime factor operating in the doctor-patient relationship, contributing to impasses that preclude the working of mutuality in general and mutual empathy in particular.

Male relational dread is a process, arising in the intensity of relationship, mostly with women. It may arise when a woman asks, "What are you feeling?" A man becomes overwhelmed by a visceral sense, in the gut, or heart, of dread. Invitation starts to seem like demand, urgency and curiosity like criticism. The more the woman comes forward, trying to explore feeling in relation, the more the man feels dread, and wants to avoid things relationally. This has particular significance for male doctors dealing with female patients.

In summary, the "normal" psychological development of men and women is profoundly different, in terms of the "being-with," grounded experiences that we would call relational. These experiences leave women feeling empathically joined and understood, with a sense of mutuality—mutual authenticity, mutual empathy, and mutual empowerment. Such relational experience may be more difficult for men to engage in, and is devalued by both men and the culture, especially in the power-over hierarchies of large medical centers.

Gender Differences in the Doctor-Patient Relationship: Three Relational Impasses

Over the past several years we have conducted workshops to bring men and women together, to address differences, work through impasses, and find creative ways to achieve mutuality in the male-female relationship. The workshops have been called "New Visions of the Female-Male Relationship: Creativity, Mutuality, and Empowerment." We have held these workshops all over the United States, in Holland, Istanbul, and China, in summer seminars on Cape Cod for therapists, in colleges and medical schools, for clergy, educators, corporations, and schoolchildren from the age of four on up. In addition, we have worked with men and women in our private practices, as well as specifically with couples. We have worked with well over a thousand people. Our thinking about gender differences and impasses is based on the data derived from this work. We have noticed three impasses that consistently arise in male-female relationships: Dread/Anger, Product/Process, and Power-over/Power-with.[17]

Dread/Anger

Male relational dread may be mobilized when a woman approaches a man emotionally, for instance, asking what he feels. A man may start to feel that nothing good can come of entering into the interaction, that it's just a matter of how bad it will be before it's over—and it will never be over. The man withdraws, the woman gets angry, the man withdraws further, the woman gets angrier.

A common example of the Dread/Anger impasse, often seen in couples, is as follows.

(A couple is sitting on a beach, relaxed and feeling close)
Woman: What are you feeling?
Man: (pause; silence; he is startled, trying to think)
Woman: Aren't you going to answer?
Man: I don't know.
Woman: Sure you do. Please talk to me? Can you tell me?
Man: Don't spoil things.
Woman: (a little angry) *I'm* spoiling things?
Man: (feeling criticized, overwhelmed with dread, withdraws, silence)
Woman: (feeling abandoned) I hate you!

What is the man's experience, in this scene? First of all, men do listen, at least until dread takes over. Second, men do have feelings and are often able to sort out what the feelings are, although this may take some time—hence the "pause." Unfortunately, women often seem to be in a different time frame, and while the man is in the midst of sorting out what he feels, she may ask again—"Can you tell me?" This makes the man feel pressured, and his "I don't know"—or even, as one man said, "I don't know—I'll tell you tomorrow"—can be an attempt at buying time to stay focused on what he feels and say it—in fact, an attempt at staying in relationship. But when the woman asks again— "Sure you do. Please talk to me?"—the man's original feeling gets mixed up with the feeling of being under pressure to respond. In this third aspect of relating, the response, things really begin to fall apart. At this point dread starts to take over, rising from the gut up, and things get increasingly fuzzy, such that feelings become blurred and homogenized into a wish to escape. At this point, even further listening becomes difficult. Note that this is not the "engulfing mother"; it is a warp in the relational context.[18] Things come to a dead stop. The relationship goes flat. The process of dread is relational, not only intrapsychic. Although there is, as always, a transferential component, relational dread is not merely a "maternal transference." Dread arises not because the woman reminds you of your mother, but because you are in a relational process in which things are happening fast and with great complexity on both sides, a dynamic in which one relational style is meeting another quite different one. At issue is the process of relationship, not the person, real or transferential. A man's dread is the result of negative learning about the process of relationship, not only in infancy but over and over throughout his life. The implications for male doctors dealing with female patients are arresting. The Dread/Anger impasse is commonly played out in the doctor-patient relationship, most often when the doctor is male and the patient female.

In one recent example, a woman with a disabled child, after many visits to her pediatrician, said to him:

> *Woman patient:* In all these visits, you only ask about her ears, or her legs, you never really ask how she's doing as a whole.
> *Male doctor:* (stiffening) I think she's doing just fine. In fact, she's kind of a miracle.
> *Woman patient:* That's good to hear. But it's so hard, I mean for me too. I need you to be there for me, as well as her.
> *Male doctor:* I'm here to take care of your child, not to take care of you.
> *Woman:* (astonished) I can't believe you're saying that. This is a very difficult situation—I need some help.
> *Male doctor:* If you don't like the way I'm handling you, I can recommend you see someone else.

The woman was devastated by these words and went home in tears. Later that night, the doctor called her and apologized. She told us that while she felt he really wanted to be *able* to be there for her, he didn't really know how, for despite his best intentions, the pattern repeated itself, until she finally did seek another pediatrician.

This, we would suggest, is an example of a Dread/Anger impasse. The physician, despite all of his training and all of his good will, is unable to break through the impasse to any kind of mutuality in the relationship.

What is the doctor's experience, in this interaction? Men report that their experience of dread has many elements:

1. *Inevitability of disaster*: nothing good can come of my going into this, it's just a question of how bad it will be before it's over;
2. *Timelessness*: it will never be over;
3. *Damage*: the damage will be immense, and irreparable;
4. *Closeness*: the closer I feel to the woman, the more intense my dread becomes;
5. *Precariousness*: even if it starts to dissipate, clear, and feel better, it can turn at any moment back to dread, betraying me;
6. *Process*: it is a shifting terrain, a movement in relationship with few fixed landmarks, a way of being in which I, a man, am unsure;

7. *Guilt*: I'm not enough; no matter what I do I can't be enough for her;
8. *Denial of and fear of aggression*: if I'm trapped, pushed too far, and unable to withdraw or leave, I might panic and hurt someone;
9. *Incompetence and shame*: all my life I've been taught I've got to be competent in the world, and I don't feel competent at this, and I am ashamed;
10. *Paralysis*: as each of these things comes up, my dread is redoubled; trying to fix things, I fumble things even more.

Note that as each of these aspects of the sense of relational dread appears, a doctor can take action to disconnect from the relationship and assert his or her authority and power, as a way of not feeling incompetent, vulnerable, guilty, ashamed, or paralyzed. Note also that the way through this impasse is not to teach medical students how to "nod their heads" and say, in an empathic tone, "uh huh," nor is it by teaching them how better to "communicate." The way through it, rather, is by addressing the impasse as a *relational* matter, based on gender differences, and understanding that it is shared, in common with other men. It is a relearning based on the early experience that men (and some women) have with their mothers (and sometimes fathers): how to be in the process of relationship with another person, and grow in connection.

For women dealing with men, it may be surprising to learn about the different relational style and time sense that men have, that is, that it may take a man longer to "process" his feelings and respond, that silence does not mean rejection, but something else. For example, one question women always have about men is "Why are they so silent?" We learned that men, when they feel that there is something wrong in a relationship, if they don't feel they can *fix* it, will not even acknowledge it at all, and will remain silent. A man offering a solution, a way to fix it, can in fact be disempowering to a woman. One of the ways out of this particular impasse is to show men that they don't have to "fix" it, but can just stay present in the conflict. As one man said, after learning that all his attempts to provide solutions were getting in the way of the process of understanding and connecting, "If you can't fix it, it isn't broken. All you have to do is listen."

Again, doctors are trained to "do" things. Although this may be true of those engaged in the more "invasive" areas of medicine, like surgery, it is not the primary focus of many other branches of medicine. Studies show that 80 percent of those coming into general practitioners' offices suffer from psychosomatic complaints, where the "doing" is to provide an empathic ear. One of the "Laws" in the novel *The House of God* was, "The delivery of medical care is to do as much nothing as possible."[19] Although this is an exaggeration, there is a grain of truth to it: the only interns who got into trouble in harming patients in the novel were those who invaded the body mindlessly, often to prove that they were real "men."

Product/Process Impasse

A Product/Process impasse occurs when the woman wants to keep opening up the process, while the man is trying to complete the task. One couple related a conversation they had when they were moving to a new house, carrying a last box to the car:

Woman: It's sad to say goodbye to this house.
Man: Yeah, but think about where we're going.
Woman: (slows down, starts to cry)
Man: Uh-oh!
Woman: Please—can we talk?
Man: Not now! We've got to finish this.
Woman: I really need to talk. I need to know where you are.
Man: (exasperated) I'm right here. Moving. How can we talk when we're trying to move?
Woman: How can you just go about moving without any feeling?[20]

This impasse, too, is quite common in the relationship between a male doctor and a female patient. A couple had adopted a baby at birth, and were worried about what they started to feel was slow development. They suggested this to their male pediatrician several times, and he at first reassured them. Finally he ordered a CAT scan. The results of the scan came back, and he called the woman at home.

Male doctor: The CAT scan came back abnormal.
Woman patient: What? How?
Male doctor: There are some calcifications on the scan. I think you better see the neurologist. He's here on Thursdays. I'll put you through to his secretary.
Woman patient: But what's wrong? What are you telling me?
Male doctor: I'm not sure, myself. There are some abnormalities, and the neurologist will be better able to tell you than I.
(Dazed, the woman hung up. Her husband came home, and she told him the news. He was devastated and enraged, and called the doctor back.)
Male patient: You can't just do that to us! You just told us that our baby is brain-damaged, and then hung up? We need to *talk* about this!
Male doctor: I don't have the time right now, but if you'd like to make an appointment—
Male patient: You damn well better talk now, or else!

It turned out that the male patient had connections with the president of the HMO, and, sure enough, soon the pediatrician called back and suggested they come in that evening, which they did. He then took the time to answer their questions. When they did get to see the neurologist the next day, the pediatrician was waiting for them in the waiting room.

The impasse here is complex, with elements of all three impasses (the other two being Dread/Anger and Power-over/Power-with), but one of the elements is Product/Process, the rushed pediatrician wanting to "turf" the difficult situation somewhere else, to complete the project and finish the product. Only when authority was brought in did he comply. The pediatrician probably had a sense of dread about opening up a deeply agonizing connectional moment with the mother, compounded by his discomfort and sense of disempowerment at not having the "protection" of his expertise and competence, since he was not a neurologist.

This Product/Process impasse is commonly seen when a doctor feels more comfortable in writing a prescription or doing a procedure rather than in talking about the issue at hand. If the choice is between competence in the "active," "fix-it," or strictly defined "medical" arena, on the one hand, and incompetence in the relational arena, on the other, the former will often win out.

Another example was related to us by a medical intern. She had a patient in intensive care who was dying, and she had made genuine connections with the family members, who had agreed not to continue any heroic measures. One night the patient decompensated, and it was implicit that the respirator support should be discontinued. The intern found that she was in turmoil about actually doing this, and went to her resident, whom she had always found to be an empathic, caring, sensitive man, despite the brutal power-over system in which they both worked. She told him her dilemma, and he said: "Fine, I'll do it."

Before she could say anything, he had gone and done it. Despite all his sensitivity, despite his being, in many ways, a terrific doctor, he hadn't realized that the issue wasn't "doing it," it was "being in her process with her." If he had been there, she would have been able to "do it" herself. Such a way of "being with another in a process," or "growing in connection," never came to his awareness.

Power-over/Power-with Impasse

In the Power-over/Power-with impasse, the man experiences conflict as a threat or an attempt to control, while the woman tries to get everyone's voice heard and attended to and retreats from what seem like definitive stands. An example, based on one medical student's dilemma, brought up in a workshop, concerns something as simple as going to dinner:

Woman: Where shall we go to dinner?
Man: Let's go to Miguel's.
Woman: How about Pentimento?
Man: Okay, let's go to Pentimento.
Woman: But it sounded like you wanted to go to Miguel's.
Man: No, no, it's okay—let's go where *you* want to go.
Woman: But I want to go where you want to go too. (pause) Why don't you want to go to Pentimento?
Man: I just want to decide.
Woman: We're deciding.
Man: We're not getting anywhere.
Woman: (screaming) Why are you yelling at me?
Man: (screaming) I'm not yelling![21]

In any Power-over hierarchy, someone always has power over you, and you always have power over someone else. In the CAT-scan example, the man's power got the doctor to face the music. Power differentials are inherent in the male doctor–female patient encounter. Power-over systems are such that it is often the case that the members of the dominant group (in this case, first doctors, and then male doctors, and, often, white male doctors) are blind to the experience of the members of the subordinate group (in this case, first patients, then women patients). Often it is only when doctors are put in the position of being patients that they start to understand, that the invisible power structures become visible. Attending to the experience of women patients is not only difficult, but difficult because the experience is mostly invisible.

As already mentioned, impasses over different ways of handling power have deep developmental roots, as well as grave implications for the nature of empathic knowledge in clinical medicine. For example, a woman patient may be told she needs an operation, and while she may not want to get a second opinion, she does want to share the decision-making process with her doctor.

Woman patient: Can we talk further about it?
Male doctor: I've given you all the information, on both sides. It's your decision.
Woman patient: But I'd like to talk more about it, I mean *with* you.

Male doctor: I can't make the decision *for* you.
Woman patient: I'm not asking you to do that.
Male doctor: I've given you the data, and now you have to decide.

The power-over structures of the society are tilted toward either/or kinds of thinking: either the patient makes the decision or the doctor does—the decision is rarely mutual. This in part comes from the male doctor's feeling that such a participation would somehow take away his authority and in part from his practical concern about malpractice. But deep down, the difficulties are rooted in the male-female impasse, where power for a male is often a zero-sum game: if I give it up, you get it (witness the Clarence Thomas–Anita Hill hearings); for the female, shared power empowers all. Strict lines of authority preclude real process work. If mutuality is a quality of the vital movement of relationship, power structures based on authority and domination over others are doomed, in terms of providing a healing environment, where mutual empathic relationships can work between doctors and patients.

Women Doctors with Male Patients

Although women's development may make it easier for them to participate in medical training with a more empathic stance toward patients, over the years in the educational system, much of the power of the "role" of the doctor clouds the empathic response. Observation of third-year students in a seminar at Harvard Medical School on "patient-doctor" communication, reveals how many students, male and female, go in a single year from an open, curious, idealistic, basically empathic and caring stance with patients to a stance that is guarded, defensive, distant, and even bitter. Fourth-year students can almost be distinguished from third-year students on sight. But women often have a harder time than men in moving through this brutal transition, for the women may feel and discuss more openly how "becoming a doctor seems to be going against my nature."

Getting to Mutual in the Doctor-Patient Relationship

Given these impasses, what can we do to break through them to mutuality—mutual empathy, mutual empowerment, and mutual authenticity?

First, recognize and name the impasses. Second, point out invisibilities in the impasses. For example, in our workshops we notice that in terms of relationship, men and women do not perceive things that may be quite important to the other gender. Invisible to men may be the "relational context" of a particular feeling or action. For instance, while "objectivity" and "decisiveness" may be strengths, they may also be weaknesses, depending on how they are used in relationship. Women carry this notion of "it depends on the relational context" much more consciously.

Also invisible to men may be the way that the attention, in any cross-gender interaction, often focuses on the men's experience. Women show a great deal of curiosity about men's experience, and men show much less about women's. This has implications for power: who has the power in a particular interaction may come down to whose experience is being attended to in that interaction.

Invisible to women (and to men to some extent) is the different emotional time in which men operate. Women tend to be much faster than men in identifying and responding in feeling ways. Gender difference in relational time must be attended to, if the impasse is to be broken through. Women are also more capable of thinking of more than one thing at a time, and this awareness will also help in the doctor-patient relationship.

Third, "put yourself in the other person's shoes." One way to teach empathy, in medical school or elsewhere, is to constantly ask the question, "What would it be like if I were in the patient's shoes?" In one seminar, for example, after a heated discussion about whether or not it would be proper for a doctor to prescribe pills to a patient with a terminal illness who wanted to kill herself, one student said, "I would never do that, write a prescription for someone to kill themselves, never." One of us asked, "If you were in that situation, would you write a prescription for yourself?" This shifted the discussion markedly. To keep this perspective throughout medical school can be remarkably helpful.

The Stone Center model suggests the *mutuality* of empathy, that you cannot be with the other's experience unless you are open and touched by others in your own experience. Mutual empathy, then, is a free flow of shared experience. A person cannot be truly empathic unless s/he has access to his or her own feelings, and that is difficult unless someone is with that person in his or her own experience. Chuck, an intern in *The House of God*, puts it, "How can you be with patients, man, if'n nobody is with you?"

Finally, form gender groups to work on "difference." The current climate of fear of stereotyping has made it more difficult to address differences between genders and among races and ethnic groups. We have found that workshops to bring men and women together to study differences in gender are remarkably powerful in teaching both men and women about empathy. First, the men spend time talking with men, and the women with women. Later, when the men and women face each other across the room, impasses develop. Through the group's process of working together, the shift takes place from isolation to connection, from aloneness to mutuality. We believe strongly that empathy can be taught and learned, and that it might best be learned not by denying difference but by encountering it.

Notes

1. Originally, this model was derived largely from experiences with white, middle-class Americans. In recent years, however, we have expanded our research to explore its appropriateness for other racial, ethnic, and/or social cohorts. Jean Baker Miller, *Toward a New Psychology of Women*, 2nd ed. (1976; Boston: Beacon Press, 1986).

2. J. Jordan, S. Kaplan, J. Miller, I. Stiver, and J. Surrey, *Women's Growth in Connection: Writings from the Stone Center* (New York: Guilford Press, 1991); Jean Baker Miller, "What Do We Mean by Relationships?" Work in Progress no. 22, Stone Center Working Paper Series, 1986, Wellesley, Mass.; Janet Surrey, "The Self-in-Relation: A Theory of Women's Development," Work in Progress no. 13, Stone Center Working Paper Series, 1985, Wellesley, Mass.

3. Carol Gilligan, *In a Different Voice: Psychological Theory and Women's Development* (Cambridge, Mass.: Harvard University Press, 1982); C. Gilligan, N. Lyons, and T. Hanmer, eds., *Making Connections: The Relational Worlds of Adolescent Girls at Emma Willard School* (Troy, N. Y.: Emma Willard School, 1989).

4. Surrey, "The Self-in-Relation."

5. Ibid.

6. Heinz Kohut, *The Analysis of the Self* (New York: International Universities Press, 1971); D. W. Winnicott, *The Maturational Processes and the Facilitating Environment* (New York: International Universities Press, 1965).

7. Judith Jordan, "Women and Empathy." Work in Progress no. 2, Stone Center Working Paper Series, 1983, Wellesley, Mass.

8. Jordan et al., *Women's Growth in Connection*.

9. Miller, *Toward a New Psychology of Women*.

10. Kohut, *Analysis of the Self*.

11. Jordan, "Women and Empathy."

12. Stephen Bergman, "Men's Psychological Development: A Relational Perspective," Work in Progress no. 48, Stone Center Working Paper Series, 1991, Wellesley, Mass.; Stephen Bergman and Janet Surrey, "The Woman-Man Relationship: Impasses and Possibilities," Work in Progress no. 55, Stone Center Working Paper Series, 1992, Wellesley, Mass.

13. David Stern, *The Interpersonal World of the Infant* (New York: Basic

Books, 1985).

14. Nancy Chodorow, *The Reproduction of Mothering: Psychoanalysis and the Sociology of Women* (Berkeley: University of California Press, 1978); Margaret Mahler, *The Psychological Birth of the Human Infant* (New York: Basic Books, 1975).

15. Bergman, "Men's Psychological Development."

16. Henry K. Silver and Anita Diehl Glicken, "Medical Student Abuse Incidence, Severity, and Significance," *JAMA* 263:4 (January 26, 1990):527–532; K. H. Sheehan, D. V. Sheehan, A. Leibowitz, and D. C. Baldwin, Jr., "A Pilot Study of Medical Student 'Abuse': Student Perceptions of Mistreatment and Misconduct in Medical School," *JAMA* 263:4 (January 26, 1990):533–537.

17. Bergman and Surrey, "The Woman-Man Relationship."

18. Miller, "What Do We Mean . . . ?"

19. Samuel Shem, *The House of God* (New York: Dell, 1979).

20. Bergman and Surrey, "The Woman-Man Relationship."

21. Ibid.

Managing Vulnerability: Power, Empowerment, and Empathy in the Clinical Setting

LUCY M. CANDIB

Reconsidering Power in the Clinical Relationship

All ways of looking at the doctor-patient interaction—whether outcome studies based on the diagnoses and procedures received by patients or linguistic microanalyses of conversation—reflect that medicine
is a practice of domination, particularly but not exclusively over women.
Most critiques define the concept of power as "power-over," or power
to dominate. First-wave feminists, accepting this view of power, were
particularly critical of the inequality of medical relationships, which
maintain gender stereotypes and leave women (and other patients)
vulnerable to abuse.[1]

More recently, feminists have developed an alternative conception of
power, the power to empower. Drawing on feminist work in fields
outside medicine, I will utilize an approach to clinical relationships in
which empowerment is the goal.

Gender influences how we view power and power relations. In qualitative studies of male and female medical students, men were more
likely to conceive of power in terms of domination whereas the women
students viewed power in terms of relationships and nurturance.[2] Nancy
Hartsock reflects, "Against power as domination over others, feminist
thinking and organizational practices express the possibility of power
as the provision of energy to others as well as self, and of reciprocal
empowerment."[3] Jean Baker Miller describes this as being "powerful in
ways that simultaneously enhance, rather than diminish the power of
others."[4] Following Baker Miller, I use the term "power to empower"
to describe the appropriate, legitimate, and necessary power of the
feminist clinician.

Self-in-relation theory, as articulated by Baker Miller and psychologists at the Stone Center at Wellesley, portrays empowerment as mutually empathic and mutually empowering.[5] Using the power to empower
others, "one simultaneously enhances the power of the other and one's
own power." The resulting mutuality serves to "empower the relationship" itself, "to create, sustain, and deepen the connections that empower."[6] Empowerment arises within the context of a relationship. "The
experience of mutual empathy and empowerment can be facilitated

through the creation of growth-promoting relational contexts in any area—the classroom, the work place, various political and social arenas, and of course, the therapeutic relationship."[7]

To define a feminist understanding of power in clinical relationships, we can turn to other unequal relationships where feminists have attempted to define the feminist practice of power: mothering, teaching, research, and psychotherapy. I cite these four locations because each of them, like medicine, is patently at risk of the abuses that result from domination or power over. Feminists have recognized that "unequal meetings"—to use Nel Noddings's term—are inevitable features of these relationships; they are searching how best to engage in relations between unequal parties to use power to strengthen the other rather than to maintain or amplify their own power.[8] I will use feminist contributions from these fields to begin answering the following questions: Given the reality of domination of patients by doctors, how can we construct an alternative practice? What would empowerment of patients mean and how does empathy contribute to the realization of its potential? Granted that patients themselves will be variously aware of and comfortable or uncomfortable with the traditional functioning of "power over" in the relationship, what does the practice of empowerment entail?

Recognition of Oppression

Empowerment must first of all entail a "commitment to understanding the world from the perspective of the socially subjugated."[9] This single statement accepts and assumes all of the realities of domination in a person's life and dedicates the doctor-patient relationship to recognizing them and not perpetuating them. The commitment to empowerment sharply distinguishes a feminist approach from other patient-centered methods that genuinely seek to identify the patient's perspective, such as the patient-centered method or the "negotiated approach to patienthood."[10] These approaches operate comfortably within ordinary medicine; they do not make the central connection between the personal experience of illness and the social structure. Howard Waitzkin writes, "The noncritical nature of medical discourse encourages clients' continued functioning in a social system that is often a major source of their personal problems."[11] In contrast, an empowerment approach requires recognizing a person's context, particularly the sources of inequality and oppression she may experience in her life, whether in her family, at her work, as a member of a minority group, or as a person disenfranchised by poverty or chronic disease.

This recognition does not make any assumption that the doctor has the power to fix the problem; rather, it acknowledges the contribution of context to her health as well as the unfairness or immorality of that oppression. The ethical commitment of the feminist practitioner must be to oppose that oppression.

I am not urging, as some critics might argue, inquiry into nonmedical areas in order to help the patient to cope, thereby "medicalizing" social problems.[12] Rather, I see the naming of social forms of oppression such as battering and racism as an essential step for a doctor and patient to make together in order to recognize where her symptoms come from and what keeps them going. When the doctor accepts and uses language that acknowledges oppression that people experience, this usage supports the reality of the patients' experience of that oppression. For instance, my asking about a black patient's experience of racism as an employee at an all-white medical center opened up for discussion at that visit (and many subsequent ones) the patient's sense that her supervisor singled her out for criticism. By bringing up racism as a concern, I was acknowledging that I knew that racism was an ever-present fact in her life. My awareness is not unique: any clinician working with women of color hears from patients about their daily encounters with racism from representatives of various bureaucracies. Of course, asking the question is not enough. Clinicians must listen for the answers and allow themselves to be affected by what they hear.

The initiation of a discussion of racism with a patient is a complex and sensitive matter. Nevertheless, given that racism is a part of the daily life of every person of color and that it takes an inevitable toll on a person's health and well-being, it is as relevant and perhaps more so than other personal attributes. In the context of an ongoing relationship, a clinician does run a risk of making mistakes in introducing the issue of racism; but over the long run failing to introduce it colludes with the dominant ideology in denying how racism denigrates and destroys people. Empathic attunement to the patient's state of mind can guide one to the least abrasive way to broach this potentially difficult subject.

The oppression women experience takes many forms, including racism, violence, sexual abuse, rape, and sexual harassment in the work place and in public as well as sexist and derogatory experiences in medical institutions. Although clinicians do not typically make the link between a woman's symptoms and social conditions, the responsibility to make this understanding overt lies with the provider. What features of context are most salient to a given woman at a given time is up to her to define when an empathetic clinician offers her the opportunity.

Requirement of Empathy

Empathy is an essential element to empowerment. Recognition of oppression describes the empowering clinician's stance toward the world; empathy describes her stance toward the patient. It includes being there with and being open to. It is a readiness to feel the other's feelings as one's own and to use that awareness for the benefit of the other. Empathy is a prerequisite for empowerment because it is through empathy that a person knows she has been heard, felt, touched. Empathy validates her experience and forges a connection with another human being.

Nel Noddings, writing about caring as a basis for moral conduct in education, includes engrossment in her definition of empathy: "I receive the other into myself, and I see and feel with the other. . . . Apprehending the other's reality, feeling what he feels as nearly as possible, is the essential part of caring from the view of the one-caring."[13] Such empathy requires inclusion, the capacity to see both from one's own and from the other's perspective. Inclusion allows the one-caring to practice confirmation: "I must see the cared-for as he is and as he might be—as he envisions his best self—in order to confirm him."[14] Empathy—incorporating engrossment and inclusion—leads to confirmation of the other and the commitment to act on his or her behalf. Thus empathy leads to empowerment because it confirms the worthiness of the other. Judith V. Jordan observes that in the psychotherapy setting the experience of receiving empathy, perhaps for the first time, can lead to the growth of much needed self-empathy in the patient.[15]

Clinicians will object that empathy as described by Jordan or Noddings cannot be practiced by a doctor or nurse practitioner with every single person in a session of fifteen or twenty minutes. I would argue that even brief interactions can be empowering. What would this entail? The ability to tune into each person where he or she was at that moment: a person here for this sore throat, a woman ready for another annual physical, a teenager with a colicky baby, a five-year-old for a kindergarten physical, a teenage brother and sister whose parents have HIV infection.

Empathy is not liking the patient, or having feelings for the patient, but does involve a real relationship between two human beings. Empathy is also an element of long-term relationships, although it need not be active at every given moment. What needs to be active is an openness to this person's experience at this time; this openness is amplified by the clinician's rich imagination familiar with the wide range of experiences and interpretations that a person might bring to the clinical encounter. The clinician uses this imagination to open up the possibility of understanding the patient's experience, without trying to limit or circumscribe that experience to some category that the doctor has already designated. Empathy enables the clinician to hear what the patient is not saying, what she is perhaps embarrassed or afraid to say. For instance, it is axiomatic that pregnant women worry about whether their baby will be normal, but the specific content of that worry varies. If I say, "Everyone worries about whether their baby will be o.k., but sometimes people have a particular thing they worry about. Is there anything you worry about especially with this baby?" I accomplish several tasks: I am saying that worrying is normal, I am acknowledging her uniqueness, and I am making it easier for her to share her concern. Questions arising from the empathetic imagination have the potential to diminish fear, isolation, and sometimes guilt. Empathy also enables the clinician to look for signs that she might have misunderstood the patient and to hear clearly when patients say that they do not feel understood.

Respect for the Person as a Person

The word "respect," like the word "caring," has been robbed of its meaning by watery trivialities about being polite. Here I use respect for the person as a person as a way to extend our consideration of personhood. One can be empathetic with an adult or child of ordinary abilities. Persons of limited abilities (who might be senile, or retarded, or otherwise disabled), however, are sometimes given a status that is less than that of a "full" person. Empathy toward them seems more difficult, perhaps irrelevant. It seems easier to be empathetic toward members of their family. Lorraine Code distinguishes the treatment of a person "as a person" from treatment "like an object," by which she means stereotyping the other.[16]

Let me offer a striking example. Some years ago our health center agreed to provide physical examinations for handicapped adults entering an independent living center. My first patient from the center was a nineteen-year-old woman with severe cerebral palsy. She was in a motorized wheelchair that she controlled with her only usable finger. I could not understand her guttural speech or her facial contortions. She could not consistently hold her head up or control her drooling. After a few desperate moments, I asked her if she knew how to use a typewriter. She managed to make me understand a "yes" answer, and I ran out of the room to locate a typewriter on a mobile stand. Pleased with my ingenuity, I stood next to her expecting some limited request. My smugness gave way to sheer awe as she painstakingly, letter by letter, tapped out with her left fourth finger the question, "What are the risks for me of taking the birth control pill?" Perhaps more than any other person, that one young woman taught me what it means to respect a person as a person.

Responding to the Changing Abilities of the Other

The requirement that the more powerful person be adaptable to the other's changing abilities is a prominent theme in feminist discussions of mothering, teaching, and therapy. It is particularly apt for medicine.

Sara Ruddick describes the quality in mothering that fosters growth and welcomes change; in response to change, a woman must be "a changing mother. . . . Change requires a kind of learning in which what one learns cannot be applied exactly, often not even by analogy, to a new situation."[17] Unlike scientific practice, which depends on repeatability, maternal thinking is based on flexibility or adaptiveness. "It is not only children who change, grow, and need help in growing; those who care for children must also change in response to changing reality."[18]

The implication of Ruddick's understanding for the doctor-patient relationship is that the doctor, like the mother, needs to develop a capacity for a constantly changing stance, both from patient to patient and in caring for the same patient across time. In doctoring, a flexible stance is essential in work with children, whose abilities change and grow so rapidly, and also in the care of people who are sick, whose ability to handle information and events fluctuates during the course of illness, sometimes leading to recovery and resumption of previous abilities, and sometimes not. For instance, over the course of two weeks a competent woman in her eighties can become acutely ill with an infected gallbladder, undergo surgery, become paranoid and delusional in the surgical intensive care unit, and then resume normal functioning in her own apartment. Such wide variation over time and across clinical conditions requires a kind of pliability or plasticity in how the clinician works with the patient and a tolerance for uncertainty about the outcome.

A patient's changing powers require that the doctor pay scrupulous attention to the person as she sees herself; and also maintain a fidelity to the person she has been in the past, and to the values that the physician herself espouses, and for which the patient may have chosen her in the first place.[19] My allegiance to the feisty independence of the woman in the surgical ICU allows me to weather a period of altered

mental ability without denying her personhood. The physician's flexible stance must transcend not only the fluctuations of illness but also
life transitions. Doctors who treat patients over many years see their
abilities change remarkably—for instance the transformation over ten
years of a thirteen-year-old girl who grows up into a twenty-three-
year-old woman. Being her doctor when she was thirteen required one
kind of attention; what she needed and expected was very different ten
years later. I needed to be able to change in response to her changes,
yet my respect for her needed to persist.

Language

The deliberate choice of empowerment as a goal, central to feminist
activities, is new to medicine. Given the understanding that language,
in both form and content, is a consistent medium through which domination is achieved and maintained, any consideration of empowerment
must address how the language of doctor-patient interaction needs to
change. Specifically, we need to examine what kind of language or
questions (since doctors' primary speech mode is questioning) might
best serve to convey the empathetic readiness just described and thus
empower patients. Following the method of a Norwegian feminist general practitioner, Kirsti Malterud, the doctor can initiate this sequence
of empathy-to-empowerment by changing the kind of questions she
poses to patients.[20] Because of well-documented forces acting on both
doctor and patient to maintain the power inequality, the doctor must
initiate this alteration in the exchange, at least at the start.

Malterud's work is an explicit application of feminist principles to
medical practice. She supports the view that language reflects the power
relations between doctor and patient; the person in charge can define
the legitimacy of knowledge and how language is perceived. The doctor (often a man) will define the "context of communication" and thereby
"reject or lose the patient's knowledge and considerations."[21] Malterud
proposes a "communicative clinical method . . . based upon the deliberate medical use of the conversation between doctor and patient."

Other analysts of medical communication have proposed changes in
doctor's language skills to enhance communication, but Malterud is
unique in defining her goal as strengthening the power of the female
patient. Her work contrasts with the model of the medical interview
that identifies attentiveness, facilitation, and collaboration as language
skills that can improve patient satisfaction.[22]

Malterud uses four key questions to strengthen the patient's power.
First, she asks for the woman's definition of her problem: "What would

you really most of all want me to do for you today?"[23] Initially, the question appears neither profound nor transformative. On the surface, it is very similar to the question, "How do you hope that I can help you" that Lazare and Eisenthal advocate for interviews with psychiatric patients.[24] The intent, however, is different. Lazare and Eisenthal see their question as providing the jumping-off place for negotiation between doctor and patient. Malterud locates in the answer to her question the distress women feel in their life situations that leads them to develop symptoms. For example, her question allows a patient to bring up a conflict between her feeling of being overwhelmed by caring responsibilities and the centrality of caring to her self-definition: "I feel dizzy when I stand up—seeing zigzags before my eyes. I wonder if there is something wrong with my brain. It might be nerves—I have been living under an enormous pressure because of health problems in my children the last twenty years. You know, that is why I exist—to take care of my children."[25]

In interviews where I have felt flummoxed by the diffuse and overwhelming nature of the patient's presenting concerns, I have found that the use of Malterud's question cuts through vagueness and sharpens the focus. Patient answers are often completely unexpected: "I'd like to try some Seldane® to see if it would help the mucus," or "Just get me out of here in time to get my laundry from the laundromat before it closes." Physician reluctance to ask the question stems from fear—fear that the answer will be so overwhelming that s/he cannot possibly respond. Noddings calls this "the legitimate dread of the proximate stranger," someone who will request more than one can conceivably give.[26]

Malterud's second question asks for the woman's view of causality: "What do you yourself think is the reason for x [the health complaints described in her own words]?" When necessary she adds: "Yes, we'll certainly find out about that—but I am sure you have been thinking about what might be the causes of x." This might be further complemented with "Since you have suffered from x in y days—you must have been thinking of its possible causes." Implicit in Malterud's repeated effort to elicit the patient's explanation is the awareness that patients' own assumption of powerlessness makes them reluctant to suggest an explanation. Initial answers such as "You're the doctor" and "That's what I came here for" are common responses patients use to deflect this question away from their ideas of causality. Persistence is well worth the trouble: the answer offers an entry into the patient's understanding of what makes her sick and opens a window onto her experience of worry. The patient will not be likely to offer a scientific explanation of what makes her ill (that her antibodies did not keep up with the virus) but scientifically verifiable causes are only a small portion of any explanation. "The patient's so-called model of illness differs most significantly from the clinician's not in terms of exotic symbolization but in terms of the anxiety to locate the social and moral meaning of the disease."[27] Being run down, under pressure, overworked, or in constant fear—the kinds of explanations patients can make—are just as valid at another level as biological explanations. Moreover, these explanations tell the clinician a great deal about what changes will be necessary for recovery.

Malterud's third question seeks the woman's expectations of the doctor's actions: "What do you think I should do about x—I'm sure you thought of that before you came here—?" As with the first question, doctors' resistance to asking this question stems from their fear of the answer. They do not want to find out what the patient wants them to do because it might be too much work; or because they might disagree with it (for instance, it might be against medical principles or it might be too expensive). Sometimes patients want administrative actions (referrals and certifications) that doctors would rather deny. Finding out the answer to this question early in an interaction allows the doctor to situate her response within the patient's expectation; or, if it is contradictory to that expectation, to open the disagreement up for discussion.

Malterud's fourth question elicits the woman's actual experiences in handling her health complaints: "What have you so far found to be the best way of managing the illness?" The question conveys the doctor's respect for the woman, and the answer validates her as an authority on her own health issues. Malterud sees her questions as using language to strengthen the patient's position and facilitate the transfer of knowledge. By asking for the patient's opinion in an open-ended way and getting her definition of the problem, these questions serve to remind the patient of her problem-solving resources and support her as a source of knowledge by acknowledging her experiences. The systematic return to her own words legitimates her use of medical language and confirms her as the expert. These steps challenge the usual conduct of the medical encounter because they imply "the existence of multiple response alternatives outside the imagination of the doctor."[28] They support and empower the patient by repeatedly legitimating her explanations, her experience, and her language, "verifying the competence claimed by her own words."[29] Malterud's method points the way toward enabling patients to reflect on their own understanding of causality and to offer their desire for clarification and naming of their symptoms, not necessarily for treatment or cure.

Laying out such an approach as a list of questions makes it appear to be a set of moves, when it is better thought of as a kind of openness, an empathetic readiness to learn, or a kind of imaginative inquiry. Yet having specific kinds of questions is helpful because together they parallel the medical model of inquiry, which is largely based on questions as the typical form of the doctor's speech:[30] both doctors and patients expect that the doctor will ask questions to explore a certain set of symptoms. In this model, doctor's questions that recognize the other's experiences of both her body and her context, that verify her use of language, that acknowledge her explanations of her symptoms, and that draw on her personal resources for problem solving—such questions can serve as first steps in making the doctor-patient relationship a source of empowerment.

Taking the Other Person Seriously

I distinguish the quality of taking the other person seriously from treating the person as a person, from empathetic readiness, and from considering the patient in her context. Taking a person seriously incorporates paying attention to where she is at the moment, respecting her fears, listening beneath her jokes, and not making light of or trivializing her concerns. Patients are concerned about how doctors will think of them; taking the patient seriously means taking into consideration what the patient might be afraid the doctor might think. Malterud gives the example of the patient who presents her symptoms as overwhelming because she is afraid the doctor will blame her for her symptoms. I am reminded of the patient who dramatically swamped me with her symptoms of sinusitis, cough, premenstrual syndrome, overweight, and itchy feet. When I asked her Malterud's key question, "What would you really most of all hope that I could do for you today," she replied with "Oh, I wish you could put me in the hospital for four days so I could quit smoking." She herself saw smoking as central to her problem, but did not want me to lecture her or blame her as she was already hypercritical of herself.

Malterud suggests two steps to show that the doctor recognizes the patient's situation: inviting mutuality humorously, thereby averting the threat of embarrassment; and allowing a dignified retreat so that the woman can be in charge of her own position. These steps, avoidance of embarrassment and dignified retreat, reverberate with the awareness among feminist researchers that what a woman says at the moment may be what she *can* say. Finding out about a woman should not be "context-stripping"; instead feminist methods "take women's experiences into account."[31]

Choice and Control

Empowerment is tied to the patient's sense of control over her life; it includes accepting her priorities, legitimating her choices, and allowing her control over as much of the circumstances of medical and health care as possible. Nurses committed to combating powerlessness can offer measures of control even to patients who are totally dependent (paralyzed and intubated).[32] To legitimate choices and to put the patient in control when s/he is terminally ill may mean accepting and supporting a patient's choices about when, where, and how to die.[33] It can also mean supporting patients in their decisions to relinquish responsibilities. For instance, a young cancer patient decides to request that the hospice worker pick up her son at school and bring him home. Although she is openly angry about no longer being able to meet him at school and jealous of the worker's health and ability to do the task instead, her empowerment lay in her deliberate choice to save some energy to be with her son when he gets home. So the acceptance and legitimation of choices to cut back or reduce activity can empower people of diminishing resources to use their energy in their own best perceived interest.

In ordinary parlance, dependence and empowerment seem to be contradictory. Self-in-relation theory offers the possibility of seeing dependency as empowering. I. P. Stiver redefines the meaning of dependency to "allow for experiencing one's self as being enhanced and empowered through the very process of counting on others for help. In these terms, dependency would be seen as normal and growth-promoting."[34] The implication of this reformulation of dependency for the doctor-patient relationship is that the mutual recognition of patients' emotional needs (dependency) can be viewed as empowering for the patient; it does not need to be seen as taking power away. This framework contrasts with the patriarchal understanding of dependency in which caring for another either deprives the one cared for of something or implies a helplessness that is seen as terrifying.

Empowerment means more than offering patients a choice. Empowerment is not just: "You can have this or you can have that; here are the advantages and disadvantages." It is a constant sizing-up activity: it is walking into a room and figuring out what could put the woman more in control, more in charge, and make her less passive. Quite often this might mean, during labor, a change in position: Would you like to get up and go to the bathroom? How about a shower? Would you like to stand for a while? Totally apart from the merits of the sitting or standing position on the progress of labor itself, repositioning the woman in labor in the upright position puts her back into the world of the living and reminds everyone present that she is a full person, not a sick and helpless patient. The idea of changing position may not come from the patient; often empowering strategies cannot come from the woman in labor because she is unaware of the possibilities or does not remember them at the time. Active listening is central. The clinician must pay attention to what is helpful and what is not helpful, and be prepared to change constantly: what is comforting at one point may become noxious and objectionable a few minutes later. Thus childbirth is one area where the clinician can promote a woman's choice and control through consciously feminist activities.

Narrative

Each woman is the keeper of her own history, the narrator of her own story. Empowerment means shaping the medical care to fit within her personal narrative. Empowerment means finding out that the woman with the fractured hip who feels inept and weak in physical therapy is the same woman who taught her daughter to walk again following polio.[35] A person's emotions and intentions are not just a momentary matter; her personal narrative has already begun and will keep on going. If we are to understand others in a "morally adequate way," we will need to attend "to how their beliefs, feelings, modes of expression, circumstances and more, arranged in characteristic ways and often spread out in time, configure into a recognizable kind of story."[36] This requires minute and specific attention to "individual embroideries and idiosyncrasies."

Mutuality

Mutuality holds a central position in feminist discussions in every discipline. Caroline Whitbeck identifies "the mutual realization of people" as the core feminist practice, typical of women's activities in teaching, raising children, and caring for the sick and dependent.[37] Mutuality begins with the practice of empathy. In clinical work, the clinician must first enter in the patient's world of experience. Jordan, with other self-in-relation therapists, sees the practice of empathy as transformative of the clinician as well. Empathy enhances both parties: "Growth occurs because as I stretch to match or understand your experience, something new is acknowledged or grows in me. . . . I am touched by your experience."[38]

Clinicians may offer mutuality to patients when they use disclosures to foster intimacy and reciprocity.[39] Responsible disclosures by doctors to patients about their personal lives derive from a relational model of the doctor-patient relationship in which mutuality is prized.[40] Likewise, feminist researchers reject the "power-over" model of investigation and insist on reciprocity as the hallmark of what research ought to be like. Ann Oakley, a sociologist who studied women having their first babies, discards the notion of the supposedly objective interview (commonplace in sociological research as well as in medicine) with "the recognition that personal involvement is more than dangerous bias—it is the condition under which people come to know each other and to admit others into their lives."[41] Researchers (and doctors) who want to know the people they are learning about must regard their work as a reciprocal project.

Clinician self-disclosure can be empowering to patients because it conveys a sense of equality between the parties. At times the patient may be entrusted with privileged information which in turn conveys respect. Nevertheless, any self-disclosures must be nonabusive and noninvasive. Such disclosures require the clinician's self-awareness and must be made for the patient's benefit.[42] The empowering potential of reciprocity does not abrogate the clinician's responsibility to safeguard the patient and establish a safe setting for the interaction.

Empowerment and Education

Giving patients information about their bodies, their illnesses, and their medications is a basic aspect of medical care. Meta-analysis of studies of patient satisfaction indicates a direct link between the amount of information physicians provide and the degree of patient satisfaction.[43] Nevertheless, doctors often relegate such teaching to others; efforts at patient education may consist only in giving clear instructions and making sure that the patient understands them. The usual approach to "education" supports conventional power relations and does not intrinsically result in empowerment of the patient. For education to result in empowerment, we must move away from the "banking" concept of education (in which material is deposited to be withdrawn later).[44] Finding out what patients already know, asking them what they want and need to know, encouraging them to ask questions[45] and enhancing their skills at managing their illness are tasks that imply a very different concept of education.

Education for critical consciousness in the medical setting requires an openness on the part of physicians about the whole medical endeavor;[46] it means allowing (but not forcing) patients into the uncertainty of medical knowledge and teaching. If a measure of doctors' power over patients is the control over uncertainty,[47] then empowerment includes letting patients in on the understanding of how little is known with certainty. Patients now know that radiation given children in the 1930s and 1940s later caused thyroid cancer, and that DES given pregnant women in the early 1950s caused genital abnormalities and cancer in their offspring. Although those treatments were given with all scientific confidence, and now are in disrepute, doctors do not present today's treatments as questionable even though they are still uncertain of their long-term effects.

Understanding patients' potential for critical consciousness allows a reconsideration of the notion of patient "compliance." Patient choices to adjust or stop medications may reflect their effort to control, regulate, or manage their own illnesses, rather than a flaunting of authority. Within their understanding of their illnesses and their medications, patients seek a way to best manage their lives, control their symptoms, and live as well as possible. For patients on long-term drug therapy, increasing, decreasing, and stopping medication are ways to gain control over symptoms and over the disease itself.[48] Clinicians can empower patients on long-term medication by expecting that they will self-regulate and inquiring into patient discoveries about their symptoms when they have done so. The facts that medication doses are arbitrarily determined, that human beings vary greatly in their metabolism of drugs of all classes, and that individuals have idiosyncratic reactions to even common drugs should render clinicians humble about patients' self-knowledge about their medications.[49]

Education for empowerment is a two-way street. A seasoned clinician will often confide that a specific patient with a chronic illness "taught me everything I know" about that illness. The idea that the patient is the teacher is not a new one, but rarely are patients directly acknowledged or rewarded for this work. In residency programs where trainees leave after three years and patients remain, the crucial role that patients play in education can be recognized both when residents leave, as part of the good-bye process, and when new residents begin. Reviewing the lineage of residents whom they have taught and the contributions they have made as individuals is a small but significant gesture that can empower patients as teachers as they begin the process once again. Some patients may be willing to tell their life story and the story of their illness in an extended narrative to a medical student once or twice a year. In our practice, we have designated these patients "Community Teachers" and have arranged a stipend for each interview as a token of respect.

Empowerment and the Placebo Effect

Traditionally placebos have been inactive treatments such as sugar pills or tangential treatments such as vitamin shots that doctors have used to help patients feel better. Usually doctors have assumed that patients should not know that the treatment was a placebo. The doctor's authority and the power of suggestion seemed a necessary part of the artifice. In other words, the practice was deceptive. More recently, doctors have acknowledged that the placebo effect works even if patients are aware that the drug is or may be inactive. Somehow the process surrounding the treatment is effective in tapping the patient's own self-healing abilities. Howard Brody attributes the liberation of the healing power to the doctor-patient relationship.[50] The next step is clearly for patients to be able to claim the placebo effect as their own. How doctors might facilitate this within the doctor-patient relationship remains unexplored.

In sum, conduct essential to empowerment includes appreciating the context from which a person comes or in which she lives (especially her oppression as a woman), taking her seriously as a person, valuing her own experience as a source of understanding about the world, hearing her narrative as it fits into her social context and into her life story, recognizing her changing abilities and potential for further change, supporting the mutuality of the relationship, and using self-disclosure on her behalf. It means opening up patient education to the uncertainty of medical diagnosis and treatment. Underlying each of these activities, essential to empowerment, is an abiding awareness of her experience at the moment, or "empathy."

The conscious choice to act in the clinical relationship as one who seeks to empower the other rather than to maintain a position of dominance begins with empathetic readiness. This state of readiness, fundamental to acts of caring, turns out to be an essential ingredient of empowerment as well.

If clinicians were to decide that empowerment made sense as a way to approach their work, how would empowerment work in a feminist practice of medicine? I will offer an extended example from a family I know well:

Josefina Santana and her daughter, Jessica. This thirty-two-year-old woman, Josefina Santana, came in bringing her fourteen-year-old daughter, Jessica, for a check-up. I have known them since the daughter was an infant. Josefina is a fully bilingual Dominican woman who works in the school system. She is an assertive woman who can be very demanding with the on-call doctor when she wants treatment for her problem of frequent urinary tract infections. In retrospect, her demands usually appear appropriate. The daughter, Jessica, is the oldest of several children. Josefina is separated from their father, who was abusive, and has a new boyfriend by whom she is newly pregnant. A few weeks before the visit I had received a request for information about Jessica from a counselor at a local family service agency. Today she sits on the examining table with her head hung down, long hair around her face; the mother immediately asks me if I want a baby sitter, tells me I can have her, I can keep her. I ask the daughter why she is there and she says, disgustedly, "for a physical."

"You don't like physicals?"

"I hate going to clinics."

"I don't blame you. And you've been to a lot of them, I bet."

I ask about the family counseling. Jessica has gone four or five times but still does not know the "lady's" name. Josefina tells me that her daughter argues with every single thing she says. I laughingly remind her that her mother said the same about her, that she still hasn't stopped arguing. "She sounds just like you!" Josefina jokingly accepts the attribution. Jessica smiles to see her mother repositioned as argumentative. I continue to deflect the mother's criticisms of the daughter and establish that Jessica is not in trouble with the law, has not skipped school, and is not pregnant. Josefina tells me when Jessica had her last period; Jessica acts embarrassed. I shoo the mother out to do the physical.

Alone with Jessica, I ask her what would she most of all like for me to do for her today. She says, "Get me off punishment." I ask her what she is being punished for. It turns out she got detention and missed a therapy session. The mother punished her by grounding her for a week, no television, and no phone calls. She is three days into it. We review that she doesn't like the therapist who "asks too many questions." Jessica is in seventh grade at junior high in the college track. She finds it easy and sometimes doesn't do her homework. She has had detention three times, once for tying another girl's sleeves behind her back, once for putting the books of a boy who had been bothering her on the windowsill where they "fell out," and once for being late for class. She does not smoke, drink, do or sell drugs, has not missed school, is not having sex and is not close to doing so. She describes constant bickering with her younger siblings. She likes to stay over at her traditional grandmother's because it is quiet, but recently her mother and her mother's companion have stopped her from staying there on weeknights because they say it is bad for her schoolwork. She likes this man and feels o.k. about her mother's pregnancy. We don't talk about her father much at this visit.

On the physical side, Jessica would like to know if I have anything for pimples. Her exam is normal. She is not particularly uncomfortable or awkward about her body. Afterwards, I go over the confidentiality of our talk, my openness to birth control when she is ready for it, and my support for her situation. I remind her that she is not a "bad" kid and has not done "bad stuff." I tell her that I think rewards work better than punishment when parents want kids to do things, and I will tell her mother that. I ask her what kinds of rewards she might like and she says, "New jeans." I ask about anything that doesn't cost money, and she says being allowed to go someplace.

When her mother comes back in, I remind her of all the really "bad" things that Jessica is not doing, and remind her that she is going to school every day, eating breakfast every day, unlike most of her peers, and not drinking a lot of soda. Mother acknowledges this all to be true. I also remind her that three detentions is not the worst thing in the world, and that Jessica doesn't like the therapist. Mother agrees that the therapist is not working out. Then comes the crucial part. Jessica is a Dominican girl in a mixed Hispanic and white junior high school. She fits in neither with the Spanish-speaking Puerto Rican kids who are likely to drop out of school nor with the white middle-class kids who see her as a Puerto Rican kid. I remind the mother that Jessica has to take "shit" from both sides, and also from any boy who tries to tease her. I remind Josefina that she doesn't believe women should take abuse from men, and she wouldn't want her daughter to take it either. She also has to remember that sometimes it is more important to defend yourself and keep your self-respect than it is to be good. Sometimes the one who defends herself gets caught when the one who provoked it does not. I redefine Jessica in terms of racial and gender issues as a child who is carving out a solid and self-respecting peer position for herself. Mother acknowledges the truth of all this. Mother knows how it is to work as a Hispanic person in an all-white school system.

After that, it is easy to talk about rewards and to reconsider the punishment strategy. At the end, the daughter throws her arms around her mother's neck and pleads to come off punishment. I sense that the mother has softened a lot. I remind Josefina that I am no better with my eight-year-old and it's a lot easier to do this kind of talking with other people's kids than with your own. I remind the daughter that her mother has forgotten a little what it's like to be fourteen. The next week, at her first prenatal appointment, the mother tells me that things are better. They went to their last therapy appointment, and she has agreed to let Jessica "go somewhere with her friends" once a week if she has no detentions.

Both mother and daughter felt confirmed after this half-hour appointment. The daughter's behavior became legitimate, even beneficial, when interpreted in the setting of gender and race; both were supported by having the quality of stubbornness in common; the mother and I shared the problem of how best to raise daughters.

This example reflects some of the elements of empowerment already described. At the same time, the vision of empowerment as I have elaborated it is open to criticism on several grounds. Critics may see it as yet another cloak for paternalism, in which apparent benevolence hides the fact that changes in language are no more than technique, a set of verbal strategies in which the doctor remains in control. Such strategies might even potentiate doctors' power over patients by making the language of empathy and support appear to be human and spontaneous features of the relationship when they are actually only linguistic devices to maintain control. Others may argue that my depiction of empowerment expands the already extensive invasion of medicine into people's lives and further extends medicine's hegemony over human activities by medicalizing problems of living.[51] The patient appears sicker in more dimensions and the doctor is rendered more powerful as a result. Finally, some critics will argue that individual empowerment will not create social change. They are right, of course. The empowerment of individuals is only a small step. And medicine is only one arena, albeit typical, of people's experience of disenfranchisement and powerlessness.

Individual efforts to reconstruct the doctor-patient relationship as empowering are fragile and tenuous in a world in which people are constantly being disempowered. Both doctors and patients are subject to being treated as objects, to being humiliated and oppressed as persons outside the clinical setting. This one relationship cannot resolve or fix all the oppression in the patient's life resulting from forces far greater than the doctor-patient relationship. One doctor alone cannot reverse the forces of authority, hierarchy, greed, racism, and sexism that patients experience. But we must dream of better possibilities. Just as we hope to raise this child to be a peacemaker in a world rejecting war, and we teach this student with the hope that she will be able to learn on her own and teach that to others, so also do we hope that an empowering relationship with this patient will free her to discover her own potential and to empower others in her life. Strategies of empowerment offer clinicians the potential to initiate, in small ways, the possibility for social change through relationships that engage, transform, and empower.

Notes

1. Boston Women's Health Book Collective, *Our Bodies Ourselves: A Book by and for Women*, 2nd ed. (New York: Simon and Schuster, 1971).

2. C. Gilligan and S. Pollak, "The Vulnerable and Invulnerable Physician," in *Mapping the Moral Domain: A Contribution of Women's Thinking to Psychological Theory*, ed. C. Gilligan, J. V. Ward, J. M. Taylor, with B. Bardige (Cambridge, Mass.: Center for the Study of Gender, Education, and Human Development, 1988), 245–262.

3. Quoted in Sandra Harding, *The Science Question in Feminism* (Ithaca, N.Y.: Cornell University Press, 1986), 149.

4. J. B. Miller, "Women and Power," in J. V. Jordan et al., *Women's Growth in Connection: Writings from the Stone Center* (New York: Guilford Press, 1991), 197–205.

5. J. B. Miller, *Toward a New Psychology of Women*, 2nd ed. (1976; Boston: Beacon Press, 1986); Jordan et al., *Women's Growth in Connection*.

6. J. L. Surrey, "Relationship and Empowerment," in Jordan et al., *Women's Growth in Connection*, 162–180.

7. Ibid., 172.

8. N. Noddings, *Caring: A Feminine Approach to Ethics and Moral Education* (Berkeley: University of California Press, 1984).

9. Harding, *The Science Question*.

10. J. B. Brown, M. A. Stewart, E. C. McCracken, I. R. McWhinney, and J. H. Levenstein, "The Patient-Centered Clinical Method. 2. Definition and Application," *Family Practice* 3 (1986):75–79; J. H. Levenstein, E. C. McCracken, I. R. McWhinney, M. A. Stewart, and J. B. Brown, "The Patient-Centered Clinical Method. 1. A Model for the Doctor-Patient Interaction in Family Medicine," *Family Practice* 3 (1986):24–30; A. Lazare and S. Eisenthal, "A Negotiated Approach to the Clinical Encounter," in *Outpatient Psychiatry: Diagnosis and Treatment*, ed. A. Lazare (Baltimore: Williams and Wilkins, 1979), 141–156.

11. Howard Waitzkin, "The Micropolitics of Medicine: A Contextual Analysis," *International Journal of Health Services* 14 (1984):344.

12. G. V. Stimson, "Social Care and the Role of the General Practitioner," *Social Science and Medicine* 11 (1977):485–490.

13. Noddings, *Caring: A Feminine Approach*, 14, 16, 19, 30.

14. Ibid., 67.

15. J. V. Jordan, "The Meaning of Mutuality," in Jordan et al., *Women's Growth in Connection*, 81–96.

16. L. Code, "Persons and Others," in *Power, Gender, Values*, ed. J. Genova (Edmonton, Alberta: Academic Printing and Publishing, 1987), 143–161.

17. S. Ruddick, "Maternal Thinking," in *Mothering: Essays in Feminist Theory*, ed. J. Trebilcot (Totowa, N.J.: Rowman & Allanheld, 1983), 218.

18. Ibid., 219.

19. Code, "Persons and Others."

20. K. Malterud, "Illness and Disease in Female Patients. I. Pitfalls and Inadequacies of Primary Health Care Classification Systems—A Theoretical Review," *Scand. J. Prim. Health Care* 5 (1987):205–209; K. Malterud, "Illness and Disease in Female Patients. II. A Study of Consultation Techniques to Improve the Exploration of Illness in General Practice." *Scand. J. Prim. Health Care* 5 (1987):211–216; K. Malterud, "The Encounter between the General Practitioner and the Female Patient—a Clinical Method," thesis summary, Bergen, Norway, 1990; K. Malterud, "How to Describe and Analyze a Clinical Communicative Method," Division of General Practice, University of Bergen, Ulriksdal, Bergen, Norway, n.d.

21. Malterud, "The Encounter," 233.

22. E. G. Mishler, J. A. Clark, J. Ingelfinger, and M. P. Simon, "The Language of Attentive Patient Care," *Journal of General Internal Medicine* 4 (1989):3225–3335.

23. Malterud, "Illness and Disease in Female Patients."

24. Lazare and Eisenthal, "A Negotiated Approach."

25. Malterud, "Illness and Disease in Female Patients," 231.

26. Ibid., 85.

27. M. T. Taussig, "Reification and the Consciousness of the Patient," *Social Science and Medicine* 14B (1980):12–14.

28. Malterud, "The Encounter," 236.

29. Ibid.

30. R. M. Frankel, "Talking in Interviews: A Dispreference for Patient-Initiated Questions in Physician-Patient Encounters," in *Studies in Ethnomethodology and Conversation Analysis*, ed. G. Psathas (Washington, D.C.: International Institute for Ethnomethodology and Conversation Analysis and University Press of America, 1990), 231–262.

31. R. D. Klein, "How to Do What We Want to Do: Thoughts about Feminist Methodology," *Theories of Women's Studies*, ed. G. Bowles and R. D. Klein (Boston: Routledge and Kegan Paul, 1983), 91, 95. Klein suggests that "faking" is part of women's survival—researchers (and doctors) need to accept it and take it seriously.

32. M. H. Boeing and C. O. Mongera, "Powerlessness in Critical Care Patients," *Dimensions of Critical Care Nursing* 8 (1989):274–279.

33. T. E. Quill, "Death and Dignity—A Case of Individualized Decision-Making," *New England Journal of Medicine* 324 (1991):691–694.

34. I. P. Stiver, "The Meanings of 'Dependency' in Female-Male Relationships," in Jordan et al., *Women's Growth in Connection*, 160.

35. Taussig, "Reification and the Consciousness."

36. M. U. Walker, "Moral Understandings: Alternative 'Epistemology' for a Feminist Ethics," *Hypatia* 4 (1989):18.

37. C. Whitbeck, "A Different Reality: Feminist Ontology," *Beyond Domination: New Perspectives on Women and Philosophy*, ed. C. C. Gould (Totowa, N.J.: Rowman & Allanheld, 1983), 64–88.

38. Jordan, "The Meaning of Mutuality," 89.

39. L. M. Candib, "What Doctors Tell about Themselves to Patients: Implications for Intimacy and Reciprocity in the Relationship," *Family Medicine* 19 (1987):23–30.

40. L. P. Carmichael, "The Family in Medicine, Process or Entity?" *Journal of Family Practice* 3 (1976):562–563; L. P. Carmichael, "A Different Way of Doctoring," *Family Medicine* 17 (1985):185–187; L. P. Carmichael, "A Relational Model in Family Practice," *Marriage and Family Review* 4 (1981):123–133.

41. A. Oakley, "Interviewing Women: A Contradiction in Terms," in *Doing Feminist Research*, ed. H. Roberts (Boston: Routledge & Kegan Paul, 1981), 58.

42. L. S. Brown, "Ethical Issues in Feminist Therapy: Selected Topics," *Psychology of Women Quarterly* 15 (1991):323–336.

43. J. A. Hall, D. L. Roter, and N. R. Katz, "Meta-Analysis of Correlates of Provider Behavior in Medical Encounters," *Medical Care* 26 (1988):657–675.

44. P. Freire, *Pedagogy of the Oppressed* (New York: Seabury Press, 1970).

45. S. Greenfield, S. Kaplan, and J. W. Ware, Jr., "Expanding Patient Involvement in Care: Effects on Patient Outcomes," *Annals of Internal Medicine* 102 (1985):520–528; S. Greenfield, S. H. Kaplan, J. E. Ware, Jr., E. M. Yano, and H. J. Frank, "Patients' Participation in Medical Care: Effects on Blood Sugar Control and Quality of Life in Diabetes," *Journal of General Internal Medicine* 3 (1988):448–457.

46. S. K. Lindemann and E. L. Oliver, "Consciousness, Liberation, and Health Delivery Systems," *Journal of Medicine and Philosophy* 7 (1982):135–152.

47. H. Waitzkin and J. D. Stoeckle, "The Communication of Information about Illness: Clinical, Sociological, and Methodological Considerations," *Advances in Psychosomatic Medicine* 8 (1972):180–215.

48. P. Conrad, "The Noncompliant Patient in Search of Autonomy," *Hastings Center Report* 17:4 (1987):15–17.

49. A. Herxheimer, "How Much Drug in the Tablet?" *Lancet* 337 (1991):346–348.

50. H. Brody, "The Lie That Heals: The Ethics of Giving Placebos," *Annals of Internal Medicine* 11 (1982):112–118.

51. G. V. Stimson, "Social Care and the Role of the General Practitioner,"

Social Science and Medicine 11 (1977):485–490; William Arney, *Power and the Profession of Obstetrics* (Chicago: University of Chicago Press, 1982); I. Illich, *Medical Nemesis: The Expropriation of Health* (New York: Pantheon Books, 1976); Howard Waitzkin, "A Critical Theory of Medical Discourse: Ideology, Social Control, and the Processing of Social Context in Medical Encounters," *Journal of Health and Social Behavior* 30 (1989):220–239.

Novelist and Character, Doctor and Patient

The Professional Understanding of Other People's Lives

When I was a medical student, working in an emergency room, the emergency medical technicians brought in a young woman who had attempted suicide. It was a serious attempt, and very nearly successful. In the emergency room, a nasogastric tube was immediately put down, the woman's stomach was repeatedly lavaged, large-bore IV's were inserted into both of her arms, and ultimately she went off to the intensive care unit. The reason that I remember this particular patient was because of the history that the EMTs gave: she's a doctor, they said, as they turned her over to the emergency room staff. And they named the distinguished Boston hospital where she worked.

I am not, have never been, inclined toward suicide. But to find myself working over a body about the same age as my own, the body of a woman who was successful in my own chosen profession, who had been reduced to such despair that she had tried to end her life—how could this not shake my foundations? I could not help thinking, as I helpfully pulled back on the big syringe, aspirating the contents of her stomach, of what might have driven her to this, of pressures which might someday drive me, or my close friends, to despair, to madness, to self-destruction. And all the other doctors in the emergency room were similarly affected, most especially the women; you could tell from the nervous comments made over and over as we discussed the case, as we tried to keep to the medical details, the issues of diagnosis and management. This patient was too familiar, too close to home; we were handling the blood and body fluids of someone who was too exactly one of our own.

The nitty-gritty detail of being a doctor requires a certain amount of detachment. You cannot put down a nasogastric tube if you are imagining too graphically the passage of that tube into your own throat; if you're busy gagging, you don't have a steady hand. You can appreciate invasive medical procedures, understanding them from the point of view of skill or from the point of view of important information to be gained—but for the most part you don't actually let yourself think too specifically about how it feels to the patient being invaded, how it would feel if it were you. And similarly, you may sympathize with patients and their families, may mourn their losses and grieve their sorrows, but you do not actually let yourself feel the pain of losing a parent (or a spouse, or a child) each time you comfort someone who has suffered that loss.

No, you keep yourself detached. You protect yourself. And though that need for protection may be strongest when the patient matches you (or your parent, or your spouse, or your child) in some specific evocative detail, the fact is that our common humanity is a pretty good match all by itself. The patients you see, however different they may be from you and yours, steadily remind you of the frailties of the flesh, of the thinness of the line between normal life and tragedy.

The limits of empathy are found in identification. The physician who would practice with sensitivity, with true compassion, with a flexibility that allows her to tailor her actions to the patient's individual needs and goals, must possess, as part of her professional abilities, a certain skill at entering into other lives. *What does it feel like to be you?* has to be one of the unspoken agendas driving the history and physical. And the understood assumption, *what is happening to you could be happening to me,* helps drive that agenda, permits the doctor to use her own human condition as a starting point for understanding other human beings. If a doctor retreats behind the protective wall of complete denial, *we are different, you and I, and what is happening to you could never, never happen to me,* it is much less likely that she will achieve any real understanding of her patient as an individual. In every doctor-patient contact, therefore, the doctor must participate in a certain construction of the patient as patient, and also in the complementary self-construction of the doctor as doctor. Although such a process of differentiation must depend on some complicity between doctor and patient, it is often the doctor who holds the dominant position within the clinical discourse.

If, however, because of certain disconcerting parallels, the doctor refrains from differentiation, and takes that final step toward identification—*what is happening to you is happening to me*—it is more likely to destroy the physician than to help the patient. You cannot practice medicine if you experience each pain, each disaster, each death, with the patient and as the patient. One may consider by analogy the case of the opera singer who must take the leading role in a profoundly emotional tragic drama while at the same time maintaining perfect disciplinary control over her vocal cords. It goes without saying that the singer who actually breaks down and cries at the supremely tragic moment—say, the second act aria in Puccini's *Tosca*, "Vissi d'arte"—will not succeed in singing the aria; at the same time if she remains emotionally immune to the heroine's tragedy she will be able to sing the aria, but is unlikely to succeed in moving the audience. The diva's dilemma is to perform the part fully while reserving total control over her vocal cords; the doctor's dilemma is not necessarily one of performance, but nevertheless one of roles (in medical school the doctor-in-training may actually find herself asked to perform the part of the patient). The doctor must engage in the discourse of differentiation that permits her self-construction as a doctor.

That self-construction is what we call professionalism. People whose jobs regularly bring them into close contact with suffering must find a way to respond with compassion, imagination, and empathy, but they must respond as professionals, and not as friends or family. By protecting yourself at some final, personal level, by preserving a carefully bounded detachment, you offer the help and comfort of someone whose job is to help and comfort, and you also preserve yourself, preserve the possibility of returning to the job again and again, day after day, year after year, patient after patient.

But how to structure this professionalism? How to incorporate the stories and the sufferings of others into your life, respect them and distinguish them, but still keep yourself protected? The physician's methodology, the technique of the history and physical, the language of hospital discourse, all contribute to both sides of this equation—they are the tools that you use to understand other lives, but still keep them at a certain remove from your own. In the understanding of the patient's story, of the life behind the story, the doctor's skills of projection and identification are essential; in the retelling of that story, the translation into medical language, that same doctor strives for professional distance and an often illusory sense of control and order.

Consider this for a basic set-up. A six-month-old male infant has an unusually cranky day. He starts out in the morning just a little fussier than usual, doesn't seem too hungry, feels maybe a little warm to his mother's touch. Then he naps for a while, but wakes up downright miserable, and nothing really comforts him. And finally, by mid-afternoon, he is screaming and screaming and screaming. His mother brings him to the emergency room.

The baby cannot tell his story. He has no words. If the patient is to be the text, then the first reading of this text is his mother's, as she tries to explain to the doctor exactly why she has been so worried. And so the first formal narrative is given by the mother, the eyewitness, prompted by the professional questions of the physician.

The first narrative goes something like this: He was just fine yesterday, and he slept through the night, just like always, and now today he's just seemed miserable all day. Not his usual self at all, crying and screaming and not eating, and maybe it's nothing, but I've never seen him like this. No, he's never been sick before, never had anything wrong with him. Yes, maybe he did have a little fever this morning—no, I didn't take his temperature, but I thought he felt hot. No, he hasn't thrown up, hasn't had any diarrhea. Yes, maybe he has been pulling up his legs while he cries.

The physician, of course, is checking off possibilities in her mind; there is some rhyme or reason to her questions, as she considers the list of things that might make a six-month-old especially cranky. Ear infection, meningitis, appendicitis. A tiny baby hair wrapped tightly around a finger or a toe. An eyelash in the eye. And the baby cries, uncomforted, through the whole interview.

A standard medical joke about pediatrics is that much of what we do is "veterinary medicine." When you care for adults, your patients bring to the medical encounter adult vocabularies and adult memories of their long and complicated lives, adult anxieties about what their symptoms really mean, the whole baggage of adult connotations attached to health and illness, disability and danger. When your patient is a six-month-old, crying about something or other, you get very little guidance. All the complex coding of medical questioning goes by the board (is the pain sharp or dull, steady or throbbing, local or radiating?), and you are left trying to make simple distinctions: sick versus not-too-sick; cranky versus in pain.

The baby's original complaint, that is to say, his screaming, his crankiness, is without words and without complexity of motive. He *is* his pain, his misery, and he screams because it hurts, screams to draw attention to his situation. The mother, in telling the story of her child and what has happened, is also looking for help, and is probably identifying herself with her child's distress; it hurts her to see him in pain, and also, after tending a screaming child for hours and hours, she is somewhat worn and miserable herself. She may also, in picking and choosing her words, be guided by some impulse to demonstrate that she has done everything that could be done, that the baby is well loved and properly cared for. Depending on her past experiences with the medical system or on her personality in general, she may be defending herself on the one hand against an imagined accusation that she should have brought the child in sooner or, on the other hand, against an imagined reproof for wasting the doctor's time with a child who isn't really sick.

It is now this doctor's job to create a medical narrative out of this baby's "presentation," using the mother's story and the baby's physical examination to create the opening episode of a medical story that will compel and propel the next turns of plot; in other words, the doctor must compose a narrative that will direct the next steps of the baby's care. She takes the various pieces of information and assembles them into medical formalism. "Six-month-old white male with inconsolable crying times one day, question of tactile temperature. The baby was formerly the 7 pound 4 ounce product of a full-term gestation, uncomplicated pregnancy, labor, delivery, immunizations up to date, no previous illnesses." And so on. (Naturally, if she is writing this down, it becomes further encoded into acronyms and initials, ever more distant from the mother's original reportage—and from the miserable howls of the patient himself.)

This medical narrative may be full of signal words. The doctor has come to some kind of conclusion, and she can foreshadow the plot developments to come by inserting words that call forth those particular developments. "Irritable," "inconsolable," for example—these are words which probably mean that the doctor has decided a lumbar puncture is necessary, to rule out meningitis. Like the mother, the doctor may try in her account to ward off ("prophylax" would be the inevitable medical word) certain accusations. She will be explaining why she was so invasive, why she stuck a needle in the baby's spine— or, alternatively, why she let this one go home without any tests at all. For example, if a lumbar puncture is not warranted, the prudent physician will content herself with describing the baby as "cranky." If she has decided that she is most worried about the baby's abdomen, she may emphasize in her own narrative that the mother reports the baby has been pulling up his legs and screaming, may report his last bowel movement in detail. If she has decided that the baby's discomfort is largely due to a red and inflamed diaper rash, however, she may deemphasize the pulling-his-legs-up history. In any case, she has edited out the intensity of the baby's distress and also the mother's, has turned those hours of crying into a point on a scale (cranky versus irritable versus inconsolable). Instead of identifying herself with the mother's distress, she has used that distress as a diagnostic tool, making various judgments during the interview as to the mother's good sense, experience, and threshold of alarm.

Just as there are many shades of predictive meaning to consider in the medical story of this encounter, there are many possible directions for this medical narrative to take. This baby could be examined by a surgeon, and would be, if the abdomen was the major concern. He could go to the operating room—appendicitis is notoriously difficult to diagnose in infants. He could have a barium enema done to see whether a portion of his intestines has intussuscepted, folded back on itself. Then again he could have that spinal tap done, and have his blood and urine sampled as well, looking for infection, and maybe get some antibiotics. Or he could be given a prescription for amoxicillin for his ear infection, or have his diaper rash annointed with an over-the-counter cream.

The baby's message to the world. The mother's understanding of the baby. The mother's messages to the doctor. The doctor's messages to her colleagues. Words and meanings pass back and forth as the initially wordless message of distress is translated, transmitted, and translated yet again. This relatively straightforward emergency room encounter is abundant in its multiplicity of narratives. It does not lend itself to any simple dialectic of text and interpretation, but is instead worthy of consideration precisely for its shifting perspectives and fundamental instabilities of meaning.

So let us turn away from the story as it happens, and consider the story as it is told, the language of the telling, and the prerogatives of authorship. Kathryn Hunter discusses the metaphor of the patient as text. She suggests that rather than viewing the physician as the author of that text, a construction that patronizes the patient and arrogantly elevates the physician to an active and even starring role in everyone else's story, the physician should be considered to play a role analogous to that of a literary critic, a sophisticated interpreter rather than an author.[1]

We find our general metaphors where we can, we extend familiar usages into less familiar territory in order to claim it and understand it. I am less familiar with the sensations of the literary critic, approaching a new text with a lifetime's worth of interpretive skills; instead, I find myself returning to the connections between physician and author, and I would like to consider certain skills necessary to both the physician and the writer, certain tricks and shortcuts both may learn to employ, and certain common satisfactions.

If the patient is the text, the physician is not the author of that text; it is, however, possible to look at the medical encounter as a series of overlapping, or layered, texts. Instead of searching for a single author, or even an identifiable collaborative authorship, there may be something to be learned from an appreciation of the different, distinct texts, the patient's "history," the doctor's "presentation" and "write-up." These interwoven stories take us from text to texture and invite us to consider the specifics of physician authorial presence. And these specifics will return us again to the issue of self-constructed professionalism; the changes that a story undergoes as it is translated from patient to doctor serve a variety of medical needs, among which may be the doctor's need for detachment, for understanding without identification.

Although there have been many physicians who have also written fiction, and some of them have been quite distinguished as authors, doctors are not, as a group, renowned for their ability to tell stories well and comprehensibly. As a group we are considered notoriously poor communicators, tending toward awkward locutions and incomprehensible jargon, symbolically distinguished in our written communications by famously illegible handwriting.

The communication of medical information follows forms and formalities; as Hunter puts it, "the aim of medical discourse is always to eliminate or control the purely personal and subjective."[2] And yet in collecting the necessary information about a patient, in successfully jumping from one line of questioning to another, in assembling the disparate pieces of someone's life into a successful narrative, the physician uses many of the professional writer's techniques.

The writer and the doctor have this in common: both are charged with a professional need (or responsibility) to understand what is going on in other people's lives and to communicate the content of those lives. And both, in order to pursue this goal, must break certain taboos, cross certain borders that are forbidden to other people.

The trait that I find most familiar from one profession to the other is this: doctors and writers are both possessed of what would be in anyone else an inappropriate, even morbid, curiosity about the tiny intimate details of other people's lives. They must both function without that dividing line that says that certain parts of life can be talked about and thought about, while others are politely ignored.

Much of the training that a medical student receives in learning clinical medicine is a training in asking personal questions. There is a very obvious analogy here to the writer of journalistic nonfiction, to the reporter trying for a professional understanding of some assigned subject, relentlessly pursuing topics that the subject might perhaps prefer to reserve as private. Journalism has much in common with the history-and-physical drill of clinical medicine; you pursue an exhaustive list of questions, reserving the agenda that informs them, you examine the physical evidence, you decide on your slant, you tell your story, assembling the punchiest details.

In writing fiction, a writer becomes responsible for the details of a character. Those details are not necessarily obtained by probing into the lives of real people, though certainly literary history is replete with such cases and with debates on the intricacies of such use and abuse. However the details are obtained, the author is responsible for knowing everything about a fictional character, even the details that do not figure in the specific fictional work. It is something like an acting exercise, or perhaps like the parlor game in Noel Coward's *Hay Fever*—the author must be able to send the character through any fictional exercise in character. Fry an egg in the manner of the character. Face a deadly disease in the manner of the character. Seduce a good-looking young man in the manner of the character. If an author's understanding of a character's range is limited to those actions actually described in the course of the book, if there is no sense that the writer knows all there is to know about these creations and could follow them through other dance steps, then the fiction usually seems trapped and limited. The author is unable to imagine other actions for the characters, and therefore the reader cannot imagine them either, and is trapped with them forever in the few sets of thoughts and sensations, encounters and unravelings for which they were conceived and to which they are dedicated. Jane Austen's characters, wrote E. M. Forster, "function all 'round, and even if her plot made greater demands on them than it does, they would still be adequate."[3]

When medical students are taught about interviewing patients, the goal is usually a global understanding of the patient, the patient's life, the patient's illness within the context of that life.[4] Even after shedding many of the elaborate trappings of the medical student history and physical (which is nortorious for taking hours to perform and too many precious minutes to describe on rounds), most physicians continue to be impelled along by curiosity. Medical training and specialization, not to mention subspecialization, can refine that curiosity into very distinct and clearly demarcated areas; it is obviously a big step from wanting to understand a man's whole life to wanting to understand the pathophysiology of his renal collecting system. And yet even the subspecialist, asking detailed questions perhaps about areas of daily life that are not usually discussed, is traveling with a figurative PRESS card, an acknowledgment of the right to ask questions, the need to be a busybody.

I would be somewhat wary of pursuing the metaphor as far as action; yes, the physician hopes to affect the lives of patients, and yes, the writer controls the lives of fictional characters, but these are very different things, and any analogy short changes both sides. (Edward Gogel and James Terry, writing about medicine as interpretation, struggle with this same issue: the physician must follow interpretation with action.[5]) After all, it is the physician's responsibility to try to understand what is going on, whether or not there is any possibility of helping. To cure sometimes, but to comfort always, doctors are taught in training, and the suggestion is that understanding must come before comforting, and even perhaps that understanding will in itself bring some comfort. It would be patronizing and more than patronizing to regard the patient as the doctor's character, belonging to the doctor, controlled by the doctor, the doctor becoming the divinity who shapes the patient's ends. Nevertheless, it is worth remembering that many writers have commented with surprise on the tendency of even fictional characters to escape in some sense from authorial control on the page. A character, once fully and properly imagined, often declares intentions and behaviors quite different from those planned by the author. And perhaps there is some metaphoric lesson in this; the physician, after all, in becoming the author of the medical narrative, the hospital story about the patient, may be assuming some narrative authority in addition to the great assumptions of medical authority. The deconstruction of the clinical text reveals that uncertainty is one of the inherent problems of medical diagnosis, but much more problematic than the ritualized uncertainty analyzed by Charles Bosk are those situations in which some certainty is assumed, and then turns out to be unwarranted.[6] If the patient does not behave as expected, as predicted, as planned for, part of the doctor's confusion may indeed reflect the loss of control over events in this narrative. That is, the doctor is faced not only with unanticipated medical events but with the public hospital awareness of those events, as they translate, beyond her control, into the various layers of hospital song and story, signifier and signified.

The six-month-old baby is still crying, still inconsolable. The doctor has examined him carefully and can find nothing abnormal on the exam. No hairs wrapped around fingers or toes, no abnormal bulging red eardrums. She has attempted, after the manner of her profession, to read his entrails; that is, his belly feels soft, she can hear normal bowel sounds, and she has put a finger into his rectum to find no masses, no internal tenderness, and some normal-looking baby excrement, with no blood in it. Of course, it's a little hard to tell on physical exam what is tender and what is not, since he screams no matter what she does, but she has convinced herself that he does not scream any more when she presses on his bowels (either from inside or from outside). She has decided he is truly irritable, truly inconsolable, not just cranky. In other words, she has decided to work him up for bacterial infection, take samples of his blood and his urine and his cerebrospinal fluid.

She explains to the mother what she wants to do, and the mother agrees, nervous and alarmed at the idea of a spinal tap, but also relieved that her worries are being taken seriously, that she is not being sent home with a diagnosis of teething. The mother waits in the examining room while the baby is taken into a procedure room for the so-called sepsis work-up. The procedures do not go particularly well. The doctor tries for some urine first by doing a bladder tap, sticking a needle in through the baby's belly, to draw urine directly out of the bladder, but it's a dry tap, no urine there. Then it takes two attempts to get the blood. And finally, with the nurse holding the baby bent efficiently into a U, it takes the doctor three tries to get the needle into the exact spot between the vertebrae and allow the spinal fluid to drip out. As it drips, doctor and nurse exchange a glance: the fluid is cloudy, not the crystal clear it should be. It looks like this baby has pus in his spinal fluid, like he has meningitis.

Now, in the secret voice of the hospital, perhaps there is a tiny whisper of "Bingo!" at this moment. After all, the correct diagnosis is being made, the correct test is being performed. Missing a meningitis, sending a child home without a spinal tap, is one of the most common nightmares of pediatrics. It is probably our analogue to the chest pain anxieties of internal medicine: lots of patients come in with faintly troubling symptoms, most don't have meningitis, but you don't want to miss the one who does. A pediatric emergency room does many, many spinal taps, and most are supposed to be negative—if most were positive, the index of suspicion for meningitis would be, by definition, too low. And so there is a tiny triumph here in a tap that is well and truly positive, in a diagnosis that has not been missed.

In a sense, the text to be interpreted has narrowed now, from the doctor's point of view. It is the spinal fluid that must be interpreted, treated, explained. There will be a gram stain to give some evidence about whether the infection is viral or bacterial, and if it is bacterial, which kind of bacterial, other tests to give a clearer picture of what is going on in the spinal fluid, and ultimately a bacterial culture, with a positive identification of the organism. Donnelly has commented on the tendency in medicine to believe that "objective happenings are more real than thoughts and feelings."[7] In this hard-to-sort-out story of a cranky baby, the abnormal spinal fluid has become the objective happening. Once the organism is known, the doctor will refer to this case not just by illness, but by causative organism: "He's the little pneumococcal meningitis who came in yesterday."

The baby will need to be admitted and treated. The doctor completes her medical narrative for the chart, documenting a long list of "pertinent negatives": no seizure activity, no vomiting. These are messages to anyone who might look at the chart that she knows what questions to ask, she knows what can happen in this disease. Her narrative thus creates a reverse template of the worst-case scenario; many of the things that could go wrong, that do go wrong in the worst cases, are here documented in their absence.

It is also the doctor's job to explain to the mother that her son has meningitis, that he will need to be admitted to the hospital for intravenous antibiotics. The mother asks sensible questions: How long? What side effects? Can I stay? And finally she asks about the aftereffects of this disease, about whether her baby will really get completely better. The doctor starts to talk about what she calls the long-term sequelae of bacterial meningitis, admits that there are occasionally problems, but emphasizes strongly that *this* baby will probably do just fine. You got him to us so fast, she says. You did all the right things.

The doctor has thus responded, both in what she writes and in what she says, to all those imagined, unspoken challenges. Her ability to project the questions of the hospital (why was this done, or not done, or not done sooner) reflects the same training that has taught her the language of her note. Her ability to anticipate the questions that may plague the mother (is it my fault, is there anything I could have done differently) reflects her sense of this case as more than a successful diagnosis on her own part, more than a medical parable with a proper beginning, middle, and end. Obviously, if the story begins and ends for her with *Streptococcus pneumoniae,* begins with the bacteria colonizing the spinal fluid, ends with the antibiotics wiping out the organism, then she fails in her ability to understand her patient (or his mother) and the significance—for them—of his disease.

What tools do we bring into medicine, how do we find ways of connecting with our patients (or their parents) at these, the most stressful moments of their lives? Books that teach medical students how to interview and examine patients stress the value of empathy and imagination to help the student establish rapport with the patient and also to advance professional and emotional growth. By listening carefully to the patient and by trying to put yourself into the situation described, you can sometimes imagine what it might be like to have a paralyzed leg or chronic diarrhea, for example, or to be raising two children, one of them sick, on a minimum wage. You can then inquire about how the person deals with certain activities or situations that would probably be difficult. Both clinical experience and reading should broaden your knowledge of groups of people different from those you already know, and you can gradually expand your more general insights."[8]

It is, however, sometimes suggested that the chief value of your personal insights is that they offer you the ability to recognize (and therefore ignore) certain biases you might otherwise fall prey to: "Self-knowledge is the key to identifying issues that might impair your objectivity as a clinician," comments one manual, advising students how to ask the particularly sensitive questions that make up a sexual history.[9] The most difficult patient to assess, however, may in fact be the patient who is most like you, whether in sexual experience or in some other highly personal detail. It is harder to remain professionally responsible, calm, objective, nonjudgmental, if you somehow feel you are caring for someone who is your own alternative self, whether the twenty-nine-year-old man who plays tennis seriously and now has cancer or the young female Boston physician who has attempted suicide.

Although all current codifications of the approach to the patient do lay heavy emphasis on understanding the patient's life, it is also generally understood that within the hospital narrative, anything beyond the biomedical facts of the case should be held in reserve for those psychosocially oriented people who are interested enough to ask. R. R. Anspach has documented, within the context of a newborn intensive care unit, the heavy emphasis placed on hard data, on lab results, on individual organs as distinct from entire patients.[10] This hospital editorial policy strongly supports the physician's impulse to tone down, remove, even forget, those same details that might promote a sometimes frightening identification.

It therefore becomes necessary to consider the uses and abuses of the various narrative forms available to the doctor. The same forms and formalisms that serve well to convey information, to establish at least the illusion of control and to protect the professional, can be bent to other, less benign agendas. Medical narrative is based in fact and tied to fact, but the doctor has a certain license, as does any author, to select and color those facts and their presentation.

What could I, as a pediatrician, do with the story of the six-month-old and his meningitis? I could tell it in the language of the hospital, of course, emphasizing physical findings and lab results, reminding myself and my colleagues, the medical students, the interns, that in a baby this young you cannot expect to find a stiff neck or the other physical evidence of meningitis. I could slant the story slightly so that my listeners would be more surprised that the tap was positive, making the baby sound less sick, making the decision to do the tap more heroic, more intuitive, a potentially life-saving piece of diagnostic medicine.

What could I do with it as a writer? I could make it into a piece of journalism, informing the general public, especially parents of young children, about meningitis and what it is and what it can look like in young children. There could be a scary moral (you never can tell!) or a reassuring moral (nowadays, this is a treatable disease) or a confusing moral (all the other diagnostic possibilities). I could, I suppose, investigate this family's life in great detail and write a piece about who they are and what this illness will do to them, about whether the parents feel guilty about some aspect of the child's illness, about how they understand what is going on and why. Or I could use it in fiction, and make the mother whoever I want her to be. It could be cheap melodrama (the parents were all set to get a divorce, but are reunited by the sudden deadly illness of their child) or studied minimalism (something is wrong in the household, but we never find out exactly what; instead, the parents make trivial brand-name-studded conversation at the baby's bedside) or anything else I want it to be. But the facts about bacterial meningitis have to be correct, no matter what I do. In journalism, of course, accuracy is paramount, but fiction also relies on a certain real-world authority. As Mary McCarthy wrote, "we not only make believe we believe a novel, but we do substantially believe it, as being continuous with real life, made of the same stuff, and the presence of fact in fiction, of dates and times and distances, is a kind of reassurance—a guarantee of credibility."[11] And so we come full circle, back to the need for facts and figures to validate the story, the same imperative that compels hospital narrative into its most rigidly scientific outlines.

And yet whatever the official hospital tone of voice, doctors have to find other routes, other ways of conversation to connect with and comfort their patients. As a pediatrician with two small children, I almost always fall back on that common experience when I am facing the parents of patients. I reach for the authority that comes from my own experience of raising children, living with children, loving children. It is a way of offering reassurance: your child is in the hands of medicine, but also in the hands of parents, who understand how you feel and what you want. I have watched numerous other pediatricians do this, in one form or another, and recognize it as a handy shortcut to declare that you know about children, you care about children.

But it is not really enough to care about children in the abstract, or to love your own children and therefore feel qualified to identify yourself with stricken parents. It is those other parents, and their children, who deserve to be at the center of the story. The officially sanctioned medical privilege of intense inquiry into other people's lives carries with it the opportunity to offer an empathy that is truly focused on those specific lives. The details of illness, health, history, and context that the physician is entitled to elicit should ideally bring understanding and a stronger sense of identification. This will not come about because the physician will necessarily discover many points in common with the patient, though those points of synchrony are valuable and helpful. With them or without them, however, the physician is allowed the professional privilege of access, and with that access, with that professional reconstruction of other lives, should come an appreciation of human variety and complex detail—which is, not at all coincidentally, also one of the great rewards of fiction.

Notes

1. Kathryn Montgomery Hunter, *Doctors' Stories: The Narrative Structure of Medical Knowledge* (Princeton: Princeton University Press, 1991), 8, 12.

2. Ibid., 52.

3. E. M. Forster, *Aspects of the Novel* (New York: Harcourt, Brace & World, 1927), 75.

4. Eric J. Cassell, *Talking with Patients*, vol. 2: *Clinical Technique* (Cambridge, Mass.: MIT Press, 1985).

5. Edward L. Gogel and James S. Terry, "Medicine as Interpretation: The Uses of Literary Metaphors and Methods," *Journal of Medicine and Philosophy* 12 (1987):205–217.

6. Charles L. Bosk, "Occupational Rituals in Patient Management," *New England Journal of Medicine* 303 (1980):71–76.

7. William J. Donnelly, "Righting the Medical Record: Transforming Chronicle into Story," *Journal of the American Medical Association* 260 (1988):823–825.

8. Barbara Bates and Robert A. Hoekelman, "Interviewing and the Health History," *A Guide to Physical Examination and History Taking*, 5th ed. (New York: Lippincott, 1991), 3.

9. Daniel Levinson, *A Guide to the Clinical Interview* (Philadelphia: W. B. Saunders, 1987), 227.

10. R. R. Anspach, "Notes on the Sociology of Medical Discourse: The Language of Case Presentation," *Journal of Health and Social Behavior* 29 (1988):357–375; William J. Donnelly, "Medical Language as Symptom: Doctor Talk in Teaching Hospitals," *Perspectives in Biology and Medicine* 30 (1986):81–94.

11. Mary McCarthy, "The Fact in Fiction," *The Humanist in the Bathtub* (New York: Signet, 1964), 186.

JULIA E. CONNELLY

Listening, Empathy, and Clinical Practice

I thought I was helping him by listening. I never imagined that one day all he told me would be helping me.

May Sarton, *As We Are Now*

Writing about the role of empathy in my life and medical practice requires that I tell stories.[1] I can tell stories from any point of view and from any level of intimacy. Stories may be about my personal and private experiences. They may explain why I feel or see a situation as I do, and therefore they may be arduous to tell. Perhaps, on occasion, I may *not* be able to share them at all, feeling the risk of sharing vulnerability, loneliness, and exposure with unknown readers to be too great. Or stories may seem to be purely professional reflections of myself at work. Still, there is the potential for scrutiny, criticism, praise, or disagreement. Tim Quill and David Hilfiker, physicians who have written stories that describe their controversial experiences, can attest to the personal risks and perhaps the benefits of storytelling.[2]

Patients, too, know that storytelling can be risky and complex. Even when confined to the assumed safety and privacy of a physician's office, the story may be difficult to tell. The symptoms may be vague and hard to characterize; worry and fear about an undiagnosed disease may leave an articulate person speechless; and uncertainty about a trusting relationship or the physician's interest may leave questions unasked and stories untold. Communication, verbal and nonverbal, between the patient and the physician affects the potential development of an empathic relationship. How well the physician listens, making the patient feel relaxed and comfortable, sets the stage for an open exchange of concerns, facilitates the telling of the story, and promotes empathy.

Here I examine listening as an essential aspect of communication and explore the impact of listening on empathy. The idea for this essay grows out of my clinical work as a physician in a rural Virginia community. Recently one of my professional colleagues commented, "Patients like you because you listen to them." I began to think about the importance of listening. Isn't listening an integral part of all patient-physician relationships? How does listening relate to empathy? Does gender influence listening and empathy? Can listening skills be developed and empathy taught?

Webster's Medical Dictionary defines empathy as "the action of understanding, being aware of, being sensitive to, and vicariously experiencing the feelings, thoughts, and experience of another."[3] Many such definitions emphasize the "cognitive response," or understanding of another's feelings.[4] We may find, however, that the emotional rather than the cognitive aspect of empathy needs emphasis. H. A. Wilmer focuses on the importance of being willing to open oneself to the experience of another person, and therefore to the emotions of the other person.[5] He writes, "Empathy involves two acts: identification with another person and awareness of one's feelings after the identification (and thus awareness of the other's feelings)." Empathy involves taking personal risks; happiness, joy, and personal satisfaction may result, but discomfort and anxiety are also possible. Usually, though, working toward empathy is worth its risks, because personal growth and understanding often occur. Last fall, an elderly woman who had crocheted a scarf for me, said to me as I stood up to leave, "I love you." And I responded, "And I love you." I smiled and chuckled to myself. I had never before said to a patient, "I love you." But I said it, in part, because she reminded me of my mother, and since my father's death (but not before), my mother and I finish every long-distance telephone conversation with "I love you." So when the elderly woman said to me, "I love you," my spontaneous comment was the same. What I felt—my warm and caring feelings—surprised me.

Another patient of mine, a counselor, told me one day while reflecting on her career, "I finally understand my therapeutic style: I listen to myself; I pay attention to what I feel when I work with another person. Then I reflect the feelings, *their feelings,* back to them." I use a similar approach when I work with patients: I listen to the voices of the interaction, listening gets me focused on this person, places my attention squarely on what is said (and not said) and how it is expressed. Slowly I begin to *see,* which means I begin to recognize what the situation is for the patient, as listening allows a broad picture to develop. Next I become aware of my feelings. Reflection is needed, however, because the emotions may arise within me or the patient, or they may result from the ongoing interaction.[6] Howard Spiro notes that empathy is "the feeling that persons or objects arouse in us as projections of our feelings and thoughts."[7] Self-awareness is very important to this process of sorting out the feeling component of any interpersonal interaction.[8]

Empathy begins with interest in the person, and the physician who actively listens demonstrates this interest from the initial moments of the interaction. "Caring to listen" demonstrates a concern and a willingness to help and to develop a potentially empathic and therapeutic relationship. Yet listening, on any given day in the office, represents a choice the physician must make. Listening is not always easy: when fatigue or personal discomfort are present, when the day is frantic with too many demands, when the patient is a long-suffering soul for whom nothing really seems to help. Listening is always a goal, but sometimes the goal is simply impossible to attain. Listening may come more easily with some patients than with others. For me, those who share experiences similar to my own—back pain, unresolved grief, loss of a parent—or those who share similar personal values, such as living a healthy lifestyle, or those patients who are willing to face problems and make changes are easier to listen to and possibly to empathize with.

Listening and Communication

Communication is the "process in which participants create and share information with one another in order to reach a mutual understanding."[9] It is an essential aspect of most relationships and is crucial for empathy. Mutual understanding is the central feature of communication in relationships: to truly understand the ideas of another person, or to be the one understood, serves to validate, to make real.

Listening is an essential aspect of language, communication, and human relationships. Everyone has the capacity to be a "listener." Hans-Georg Gadamer writes, "One who listens is fundamentally open. Without this kind of openness to one another there is no genuine human relationship. Belonging together always means being able to listen to one another."[10] Listening does not represent a "further stage" of development that must be accomplished; without listening, it may be impossible even to form relationships.

Speaking and listening are complementary. Listening may be thought of as the "flip side" or mirror-image of spoken language. But speaking holds the more valued position in our method of communication, and as G. Fiumara observes, our "system of knowledge tends to ignore listening processes."[11] Perhaps this is because listening, the receptive mode, appears to most observers as a void, a silence, an emptiness: in listening there is no sound, no obvious power, no apparent control.[12] Listening for some individuals may elicit feelings of vulnerability, loss of control, insecurity, or impatience. Much like empathy, listening requires taking risks and possible exposure to uncomfortable feelings. Yet without listening, speaking serves no purpose.[13]

In most conversations, the roles of the speaker and the listener shift back and forth. Balance is created in the exchange. In medical encounters, too, both the patient and the physician should be listeners as well as speakers. Yet one individual, the physician, is so dominant—in the vast majority of instances, the physician both opens the conversation and closes it.[14] Listening, when seen as a passive, powerless function, is not a natural role for physicians, men or women, because they are taught to take charge, to direct, and to ask specific questions as they attempt to "pinpoint the seat of the trouble."[15] H. B. Beckman and R. M. Frankel, studying seventy-four office visits, demonstrated that 69 percent of physicians listened to the patient an average of only eighteen seconds before interrupting and "taking control of the visit by asking increasingly specific, closed-ended questions" that effectively ended the flow of information.[16] Interruptions are made in an effort to be effective. Yet to be truly effective, physicians need to listen more carefully. They must diagnose the problem whether its origins are in disease, social relationships, socioeconomic distress, or lifestyle or behavioral characteristics. They must understand what the problem means or represents to the patient. They must encourage expression as a therapeutic strategy for the relief of suffering. They must understand various aspects of the patient's story[17] or, when they are fortunate, the patient's whole story.[18]

Michael Balint, a British psychoanalyst who worked with general practitioners to explore the patient-physician relationship, described two different styles of listening in patient interactions. One, the "great detective" style, is employed regularly by physicians; the second, highly recommended but less commonly used, requires "tuning in" to the patient's wavelength. This type of listening often results in a "flash" of understanding for the patient, the physician, or both.[19]

The great detective style requires that the physician listen "most intently, observe everything carefully and, if necessary, examine conscientiously every area which, in his [her] opinion, might be involved in the patient's problems. No stone must go unturned."[20] Using this method, the physician focuses on the disease rather than on the patient. If the physician focuses on diagnosing the disease, rather than on helping the patient, a situation described by R. J. Baron may result.[21] Baron writes, "It happened the other morning on rounds, as it often does, that while I was carefully ausculting a patient's chest, he began to ask me a question. 'Quiet,' I said, 'I can't hear you while I'm listening.'" Balint and Theodur Reik describe similar phenomena among physicians who listen only to the biomedical aspects of the patient's story and fail to hear what is important to the patient.[22] As Balint wrote, "If you ask questions you will get answers: and nothing else."[23] The second technique requires the doctor to "tune in," focusing his or her "attention on what it is the patient is trying to convey at that particular time."[24] This patient-centered method allows the doctor and patient to talk to each other with less possibility of a misunderstanding.[25] It aims not only to diagnose the patient's disease but also to understand what the illness or symptom means to the patient. To use this method, physicians must respond to "cues by which patients express their feelings," must be self-aware enough to respond to the patient's feelings, must "organize complex biopsychosocial information from the patient," and must practice active, attentive listening.[26]

The Voices of Listening

In his autobiography, William Carlos Williams[27] described the attention necessary to focus himself on the patient—his or her peculiarities, reticences, or candors—and on the details of the case. Attention is this ability to "tune in" to the interaction, observing nonverbal cues and listening carefully to the various speakers and voices. Nonverbal cues and styles of expression (including facial expressions, eye contact, voice qualities, and body positions and movements) contribute to the language of communication and encourage the speaker to continue.[28]

The listener's attention needs to be free enough to make observations regarding both self and speaker, but the listener must not relax. The listener must focus on the patient and listen and observe attentively, ready to choose how and when to respond. Freud defined a special kind of attention, *gleichschwebend*, which Theodur Reik translated as "free-floating" attention. Freud recognized the clinical need for this special type of attention which, once attained, can be maintained rather easily and which helps the listener avoid interpretive problems. For instance, Reik notes that "if we strain our attention to a certain point, if we begin to select from among the data offered and seize upon one fragment especially, then, Freud warns us, we follow our own expectations or inclinations. The danger naturally arises that we may never find anything but what we are prepared to find."[29]

The listener's task is remarkably complex. For instance, the physician who attempts to gain this state of patient-centered attention must observe the nonverbal cues while listening to the many voices within the ongoing dialogue: the patient's literal voice, the patient's metaphorical voice, the doctor's diagnostic voice, the doctor's great detective voice, the doctor's interpretive voice, the doctor's personal, or emotional, voice, and perhaps others. This patient-centered yet free-floating attention may be difficult to attain. Reik comments that "one gets the impression that it is a course easy to pursue. But in practice it is hardly less difficult than the course required of the patient."[30] If the physician is going to understand the patient, however, she must listen carefully to each voice as the communication with the patient proceeds and deepens.

For those inexperienced with or unaware of the voices of communication that physicians encounter and learn to recognize, an analogy can be made to the voices of reading. G. Stewart notes that "we listen while we read."[31] Although some argue that "literature is text, not talk," it does in fact "speak" to us. Reading, as it proceeds, does give way to voice. The reader on one level may simply hear the written words as they are being read. This is similar to the physician's hearing the patient literally. Or the reader's voice may ask a question to clarify the text—"What does that mean? What is the author really saying? What has been omitted?"—just as the physician wonders what the patient's words, "I just feel 'punk,' or 'dizzy,' or 'giddy-headed,'" really mean. On another level, the reader's inner voice may suggest an interpretation of the text, for example, while reading poetry. As the reading continues, associations to previously read works may be evoked, just as the physician is stimulated to recall other patients with similar presentations or stories. The reader and the physician also share the personal, often emotional, voice—that of recognition and connection—when what is read seems to express one's own experience or perception of life events.[32] Another difficult challenge involves turning off, or suspending, at least for a few moments, certain cognitive habits—translation, analysis, judgment—in order to allow the speaker's own cultural, linguistic, and social narrative to be heard freely, in its own context, in its own idiom.[33] Suspending the cognitive provides the physician with the opportunity to enter into the patient's world—to respond with empathy, to clarify, to envision that world and its impact on the person's state of health or illness.

Stories of Listening

As a third-year medical student, I learned that one must be attentive to all possibilities—free of restrictions and preconceived ideas. I stumbled upon this notion while helping care for one particular patient. She was a twenty-five-year-old with insulin-dependent diabetes mellitus who presented to the emergency room with the signs of ketoacidosis: Kussmaul's respiratory pattern, hypotension, confusion. The resident and intern circled her, beginning intravenous lines and efficiently examining her for infection: ears, lungs, abdomen, feet, urine. But no reason could be found to explain the occurrence of the ketoacidosis. Unstable or brittle diabetes was their explanation.

She had been admitted to the hospital with ketoacidosis four times in the previous six months, and each time no explanation could be found other than to say that she had brittle diabetes. Listening to myself, before I had ever talked with the patient, I heard myself asking, Why does her problem recur? Why? The medical texts all mentioned specific reasons and we had none, just "brittle diabetes," which seemed unsatisfying.

When she began to feel better, I spent some time with her. After a few days she began to speak about her life. What I remember is listening to her tell me that her marriage was not very happy, that her husband was having an affair, and that she feared losing him. She continued talking as I listened.

"When I am ill, my husband is so caring.

"The last few times I was here, we made up and for a while we had fun together.

"My insulin—you know, if I don't take it, what happens.

"So I thought maybe this time, too. . . . "

There was the "flash,"[34] the "Ah ha" of clinical medicine, the moment when the pieces of the puzzle fit and the clinical situation becomes clear. Brittle diabetes was not her problem—her marriage and her fear were. Listening was the key: listening to her and to the nagging questions within myself.

After the completion of my residency I worked for a year as an emergency room physician. In that year, I evaluated about seven thousand patients, far more than in medical school and residency training combined. Reflecting on my experience, I realized that I had become fascinated with listening to the various voices and observing differences among patients who came to the emergency room because of similar problems: chest pain, shortness of breath, abdominal pain, and so on. Sometimes simply looking at the individual with shortness of breath indicated that the problem was asthma or congestive heart failure, while, in other cases, listening to the rapid, forced, or high-pitched quality of the speech suggested that anxiety was the likely cause of the presenting symptom. But how could I be sure of the diagnosis based on such observations? Confirmation required that I listen to a story: What had happened? When had the symptoms begun and what was the context? Listening to these stories, staying tuned in, I became more certain about the diagnoses made, the treatments prescribed, and the recommendations suggested. After eight years in practice, I understand now another function of listening: that listening can be therapeutic in and of itself.

Listening: The Patient's Point of View

After many interactions with patients, I am convinced of the benefits of telling one's story, of having someone listen and try to understand. Office patients in rural Virginia often say "thanks for listening." Occasionally a day will go by when I don't examine anyone—I just listen to them and the stories they want and perhaps need to tell. Several days ago I observed an interview between a medical resident, whose goal was "just to be quiet and let the patient talk," and a patient. Prior to this session, the physician had dreaded the patient's visits to the clinic. He understood very little about her; empathy was not part of their relationship, until he really listened to her. At the close of the interview, the patient said, "Oh, I feel so much better talking to you like this. Thanks for letting me tell you everything."

Although I am a physician, I am also a patient. And as a patient I have experienced the incredible relief from despair and the comfort offered by a physician who is a good listener. My experience as a patient offers important insights to me about the world of the patient. We patients, I expect, are similar in what we need and want. Patients, both men and women, come to the office with stories to tell. We want to be listened to. As Alice Walker wrote in her novel *The Temple of My Familiar*, "really what we are looking for is someone to be able to hear us."[35] Not only do we want to be heard, "we want to be understood."[36]

A physician who is a good listener encourages and enables the patient to speak the unspeakable, to search the depths of the soul, to put voice to the unconscious. Just yesterday a patient said to me, "Yes, I enjoyed talking with you last week. I felt better, and, you know, I told you things I've never told anyone, I wouldn't dare." Another patient, Caro Spencer in May Sarton's novel *As We Are Now*, confirms this function of listening when she comments, "I imagine when I am lying here on my bed that I am talking to a wise and omniscient listener, a Doctor of Souls to whom I can say things I might not dare say to myself alone."[37] Listening helps patients tell their stories, and this telling in turn helps them discover their personal voice as they become aware of themselves, their wishes, and choices.

A good listener respects silence and feels comfortable with the inevitable discomfort of a pause in the conversation. Pauses may be used purposefully by the physician to encourage the patient to continue. At other times, what appears to be a pause may be a silence—a time when no words are needed to convey the impact or meaning of the situation. Again Caro Spencer's comments help clarify for us the importance of silence. "Sometimes silence is the greatest sign of understanding and of respect. It is far more consoling than words of false comfort." She warns the listener to avoid clichés and empty comments such as "It can't be as bad as all that" or "Things will surely be better tomorrow, dear," and she reminds us that in silent listening, there is power to heal. "True caring," as Sarton's Caro Spencer observes, does indeed "show itself in silence, by the quality of listening or some shy gesture of love."[38]

The listener may have a difficult job and tolerance may be hard to find, yet the more difficult the story, the more it needs to be told. Patients are often afraid to say what they are thinking, because they believe that their thoughts might be harmful to others. Patients often comment, "I'm glad you are here. I just didn't have anyone to talk to, anyone who would listen." Or, "It wouldn't be fair to talk with my family about that." Caro Spencer fears that the painful story of her helplessness "creates too much havoc in a listener, is too disturbing, because nothing can really be done to help us [the elderly]." Relief comes however when a caring person encourages her to talk. Caro reflects, "she did not hurry off without listening."[39] How often have I gone to the hospital to see my patients in between teaching sessions or meetings, only to hear them ask "just one more question" as I rush out the door, hoping I won't be late.

Stories, Empathy, and Gender

Our county of 21,000 people has three women physicians. When I hear stories about the old-time docs of the county, they are all about men such as William Carlos Williams's "Old Doc Rivers."[40] There were no women physicians. Patients had few, if any, choices about their physicians. When I ask women patients, new referrals to my practice, "Why did you choose me?" I frequently hear, "You are a woman." "I want a woman physician." "We are alike. We're both women." "I know you will understand another woman." Everyone wants to be understood.[41] And some women believe that they will best be understood by another woman; perhaps the parallel belief is held by men.

One week last May three patients whom I had cared for since I moved to the Virginia countryside died. One patient was in her eighties; she had fallen, injuring her head. After a week in the neurosurgical intensive care unit, she died. Watching her husband during that week, as he waited and hoped for her to respond, was difficult. Losing her made me very sad because over the years she had become a friend of sorts. She was well known in our office, and we cared about her. I stood at her bedside the day before she died with her daughter, whom I had just met. We were telling stories about her mother—the patient. I told the daughter, "Once, needing to change your mother's medication, but aware of her sensitivity about age, I said to her, 'This drug has been specially formulated for people as they get older.' She retorted, 'Well, you should receive the Nobel Prize for Tact and Diplomacy!' I laughed, but she didn't." I wrote the families of the other patients to express my sympathy to them. Often sympathy has a negative connotation in medicine as being "overly emotional or too close to the patient." Sympathy, however, serves an important role in clinical medicine because it enables physicians an opportunity to express their emotions (at least to patients' families).

During the winter I attended on the inpatient medical service. The house staff admitted a woman, who looked much older than her twenty-eight years, to our service. She was a diabetic and had been on dialysis for six years. Her skin was gray and pale, her hair oily and matted from fever, and her breath smelled from her illness. She lay in bed nearly unresponsive for several days. The general feeling on rounds was a vague repulsion: no one knew her and she looked rather frightening—so young, yet so old and so gray.

One morning, when she felt better, I asked her if I could bring the students in to talk with her. She began to tell us about her life. In her teens she had been physically abused. To avoid the pain, she occasionally quit taking her insulin. In diabetic ketoacidosis, she would be admitted to the safety and warmth of the hospital—a safety and warmth she could not find in her home. As she spoke, I looked around at the students. Their eyes were firmly fixed on hers; there was no sense of repulsiveness, no anxiousness to leave her as our image of her was enlarged and we came to understand her. She told us how she was hoping to go home in two days. Now that she was married and had children, she preferred her home to the hospital. We listened to her and we learned. I remembered the diabetic patient I had had as a third-year student and the impact of knowing her story. Now I found myself listening to another patient's story and hoping the students would learn to value empathic relationships. This patient thanked us for coming to see her and commented that she felt better, that the hospital was still a safe place for her, and that she had enjoyed talking to us.

Exactly how gender affects the listening skills is unclear. On the one hand, some women may be better listeners than men. According to some linguistic researchers, this may be because girls are taught to listen. Empathic relationships may develop more quickly with women physicians; as women, they may be more comfortable supporting others rather than "giving opinions and advice."[42] On the other hand, women may fear that developing supportive relationships may be misinterpreted as "casting them in a subordinate position"[43] and that listening imposes a personal threat of "silence."[44] M. F. Belenky, B. M. Clinchy, N. R. Goldberger, and J. M. Tarule in *Women's Ways of Knowing* describe the struggle that women experience between voice, speaking up, and silence.[45] How this struggle affects women physicians and the relationships they form is not clear. Some women may be skillful listeners because of the social roles and expectations imposed on them during childhood. For some women, however, listening may seem risky, as it places them in the vulnerable position of silence. If the problem of silence exists for the woman physician, it must be confronted, because the opportunity to tune in with the patient and to understand the patient's story appears to be too valuable to avoid.

Nonverbal cues, an integral part of listening and communication, may explain why some women prefer a woman physician. In *Nonverbal Sex Differences: Accuracy of Communication and Expressive Style*, Judith Hall summarizes, "women are better at decoding nonverbal cues, at recognizing faces, and at expressing emotions via nonverbal communications than are men." They have more "expressive faces, smile more, gaze more, employ smaller approach distances to others, and are approached closer by others. Women use body movements and positions that appear to be less restless, more expressive, more involved . . . than men."[46] These observations suggest that women physicians may appear more empathic than men. And women patients may feel more comfortable, more understood, or more accepted by women physicians who express themselves in similar ways.

Although listening may appear mundane, it has a profound impact on every patient-physician relationship. Many problems arise when listening is not a priority of the physician—understanding does not occur, empathy is compromised, the therapeutic alliance may not develop, healing is minimized, and suffering may result. Problems of caring, including ethical dilemmas and malpractice concerns[47] can arise when doctor and patient do not relate to, or understand, one another. Inequities and conflicts occur when issues important to the patient, such as patient beliefs, values, family traditions, are deflected or are not taken seriously. When a patient refuses to accept the physician's suggested or prescribed means of diagnosis or treatment and the physician does not listen to the patient's reasoning, an ethical dilemma evolves. Many of these kinds of problems can be prevented or resolved by listening to the patient.

Physicians must learn to listen not only for the disease-related information but also for information about the attribution of the symptoms, the patient's judgments about why the symptoms are occurring, and related information concerning work, family, finances, and other struggles. The capacity to listen can be developed and specific skills can be learned. For instance, when a patient says, "Doc, my back hurts so bad when I'm at work," the physician has a choice to make: the back pain must, of course, be characterized and evaluated, but the opportunity to inquire about the patient's work and life is present: Why do you think it hurts at work? Tell me about your work. How does your back pain affect your work, your life? Yet physicians, skilled as "great detectives" and focused on the biomedical approach, move to the back pain and the specific diagnosis. They in effect distance themselves from the opportunity to understand the patient.[48] This intense focus on the disease also limits their understanding of the social, cultural, and behavioral determinants of illness and disease and their opportunities for healing.

Medical students (in my experience) seem to know much more about "clinical distance" and Osler's praise for equanimity than they do about empathy.[49] Distance and balance are important. But where do students really learn about caring? How do they learn to feel comfortable in helping relationships? Medical educators and students need to answer these questions. As technology advances and threatens to increase the distance between patient and physician, the probability of becoming overly involved may be less than it was during Osler's day. Perhaps we need to reconsider our emphasis on distance and exchange it for compassion, caring, self-awareness, closeness, and empathy.

Changes in the medical school curriculum, such as the Doctor-Patient courses for first-year students,[50] educational experiences that occur in the community, and the emphasis on humanities in medicine[51] can diminish the gulf between doctors and patients. They can promote the physicians' capacities to *hear* while they are listening.

Notes

1. Epigraph: M. Sarton, *As We Are Now* (New York: W. W. Norton and Co., 1973), 7.

2. T. E. Quill, "Death and Dignity: The Case of Diane," *New England Journal of Medicine* 325 (1991):658–660; D. Hilfiker, "Facing Our Mistakes," *New England Journal of Medicine* 310 (1984):118–122.

3. *Webster's Medical Dictionary* (Springfield, Mass.: Merriam-Webster, 1986).

4. S. D. Nightingale, P. R. Yarnold, and M. S. Greenberg, "Sympathy, Empathy, and Physician Resource Utilization," *Journal of General Internal Medicine* 6 (1991):420–423.

5. H. A. Wilmer, "The Doctor-Patient Relationship and the Issues of Pity, Sympathy, and Empathy," *British Journal of Medical Psychology* 41 (1968):243–248.

6. L. J. Henderson, "Physician and Patient as a Social System," *New England Journal of Medicine* 212 (1935):819–823.

7. H. Spiro, "What Is Empathy and Can It Be Taught?" *Annals of Internal Medicine* 116 (1992):843–846.

8. M. F. Lindquist, "Physician Self-Awareness," *Communicating with Medical Patients* (Newbury Park, Calif.: Sage Publications, 1989), 64–72.

9. E. Rogers, *Diffusion of Innovations*, 3rd ed. (New York: Free Press, 1983).

10. H. G. Gadamer, *Truth and Method*, trans. W. Glen-Doepel, J. Cumming, and G. Barden (London: Sheed & Ward, 1979).

11. G. Fiumara, *The Other Side of Language: A Philosophy of Listening* (London: Routledge, 1990), 1.

12. D. Tannen, "Different Words, Different Worlds," Chapter 2 in Tanner, *You Just Don't Understand: Men and Women in Conversation* (New York: Ballantine Books, 1990).

13. Fiumara, *The Other Side of Language*, 12–15.

14. E. G. Mishler, "Routine Practice," *The Discourse of Medicine: Dialectics of Medical Interviews* (Norwood, N.J.: Ablex Publishing, 1984).

15. E. Balint and J. S. Norell, eds., *Six Minutes for the Patient: Interactions in General Practice Consultation* (London: Tavistock Publications, 1973).

16. H. B. Beckman and R. M. Frankel, "The Effect of Physician Behavior on the Collection of Data," *Annals of Internal Medicine* 101 (1984):692–696.

17. R. C. Smith and R. B. Hoppe, "The Patient's Story: Integrating the Patient- and Physician-Centered Approaches to Interviewing," *Annals of Internal Medicine* 115 (1991):470–477.

18. J. E. Connelly, "The Whole Story," *Literature and Medicine* 9 (1990):150–161.

19. M. Balint, "Research in Psychotherapy," in *Six Minutes*, ed. Balint and Norell.

20. Balint, "Research in Psychotherapy", 7.

21. R. J. Baron, "An Introduction to Medical Phenomenology: I Can't Hear You While I'm Listening," *Annals of Internal Medicine* 103 (1985):606–611.

22. M. Balint, *The Doctor, His Patient, the Illness* (London: Pitman Medical Publishing, 1964), 1–20; T. Reik, "The Workshop," in Reik, *Listening with the Third Ear* (New York: Jove Publications, 1948), 156–172.

23. Balint, *The Doctor, His Patient, the Illness*, 10.

24. Balint and Norell, eds., *Six Minutes for the Patient*, xii.

25. Balint, "Research in Psychotherapy," 8.

26. M. Stewart and D. Roter, *Communicating with Medical Patients* (Newbury Park, Calif.: Sage Publications, 1989).

27. William Carlos Williams, "The Practice," in *The Autobiography of William Carlos Williams* (New York: New Directions, 1948), 356–362.

28. C. Carson, "A Course in Nonverbal Communication for Medical Education," Rochester, N.Y., 1988.

29. Reik, "The Workshop," 156–172.

30. Ibid.

31. G. Stewart, "'To Hear with Eyes': Shakespeare as Proof Text," *Reading Voices: Literature and the Phonotext* (Berkeley: University of California Press, 1990).

32. M. White, personal communication, 1992; W. M. Zinn, "Doctors Have Feelings Too," *Journal of the American Medical Association* 259 (1988):3296–3298; Julia E. Connelly, "Emotions and the Process of Ethical Decisionmaking," *Journal of the South Carolina Medical Association* (1990):621–623.

33. M. White, personal communication, 1992.

34. Balint, "Research in Psychotherapy," 1–18; Balint and Norell, eds., *Six Minutes for the Patient,* 19–43.

35. A. Walker, *The Temple of My Familiar* (New York: Harcourt Brace Jovanovich, 1989).

36. Tannen, "Different Words, Different Worlds."

37. Sarton, *As We Are Now,* 20.

38. Ibid., 49, 74.

39. Ibid., 73.

40. William Carlos Williams, *The Doctor Stories,* comp. Robert Coles (New York: New Directions, 1984).

41. Tannen, "Different Words, Different Worlds", 131; Walker, *The Temple of My Familiar,* 187.

42. D. Tannen, "Different Words, Different Worlds", 138, 133.

43. Ibid., 139.

44. Tillie Olsen, *Silences* (New York: Dell, 1965).

45. M. F. Belenky, B. M. Clinchy, N. R. Goldberger, and J. M. Tarule, *Women's Ways of Knowing: The Development of Self, Voice, and Mind* (New York: Basic Books, 1986).

46. J. Hall, *Nonverbal Sex Differences: Accuracy of Communication and Expressive Style* (Baltimore: Johns Hopkins University Press, 1984), 1, 143.

47. V. Warren, "Feminist Directions in Medical Ethics," *Hypatia* 4 (1989):72–87.

48. Baron, "An Introduction to Medical Phenomenology", 606–611.

49. R. J. Baron, "Clinical Distance: An Empathic Rediscovery of the Known," *Journal of Medical Philosophy* 6 (1981):3–21; W. Osler, *Aequanimitas, with Other Addresses,* 2nd ed. (New York: McGraw-Hill, 1906), 2–11.

50. W. T. Branch, R. A. Arky, B. Woo, J. D. Stoeckle, D. B. Levy, and W.

C. Taylor, "Teaching Medicine as a Human Experience: A Patient-Doctor Relationship Course for Faculty and First-Year Medical Students," *Annals of Internal Medicine* 114 (1991):482–489.

51. Baron, "An Introduction to Medical Phenomenology," 606–611; R. M. Arnold, G. J. Povar, J. D. Howell, "The Humanities, Humanistic Behavior, and the Humane Physician," *Annals of Internal Medicine* 106 (1987):313–318.

SECTION FOUR

Empathy and the Politics of Difference

CAROL C. NADELSON

Health Care
Is Society Empathic with Women?

The changes that have taken place in the U.S. health care system over the last few decades challenge health care providers' ability to forge and maintain empathic connections between patients and those caring for them. Criticisms of current health care practices have focused on the need to maintain a humane health care environment in the face of encroaching technological and economic pressures. Despite these explicit concerns, however, empathy is not often accorded much attention in health policy discussions or decisions. Here I address empathy as it exists within the health care system: between doctors, patients, and the "system" itself. Using gender as an example, I will introduce and examine a concept of "societal empathy."

Empathy: Doctors, Patients, and Society

The word "empathy" has many definitions, and it is used in many ways. It is generally understood within the context of one-to-one relationships. When used synonymously, if imprecisely, with sympathy or compassion, it implies understanding, sensitivity, and an ability to provide solace and comfort.

In the psychoanalytic literature, where the concept has achieved a dominant place in recent years, it connotes an affective attunement to another.[1] Heinz Kohut views empathy as "a fundamental mode of human relatedness . . . the recognition of the self in the other . . . the accepting, confirming and understanding human echo . . . the resonance of essential human alikeness."[2] This conceptualization assumes a shared core of human awareness that enables us to connect with the inner experiences of others.

Each definition describes a connection between people that is resonant, comforting, and caring. Eric Cassell suggests, however, that "we can never truly experience another's distress."[3] "It is possible to know the suffering of others, to help them, and to relieve their distress, but never to become one with them in their torment."[4] In emphasizing that we can approximate and imagine the experiences of others without truly sharing them, he implies that there is a limit to our empathic capacities.

Being empathic has been described as "an act of will and creativity,"[5] suggesting that motivation, effort, and an active commitment are required. This is particularly important to keep in mind in a society where decisions are made through delegated authority; where those with authority may not share the life experiences or needs of those without it. Because most contemporary societal policies and priorities are predicated on the delegation of decision-making authority, we expect that those who are entrusted with this responsibility are able to be empathic with people whose experiences, values, and needs differ from theirs.

Although we all possess a capacity for empathy, we are not equally or always empathic. Often we have difficulty being empathic with people we dislike or do not respect, or with those whose values, experiences, customs, beliefs, or ideals are different from ours. We have difficulty being empathic with people whose race, sex, culture, or class differs from ours. We even have difficulty being empathic with those who suffer from certain illnesses, such as AIDS, alcoholism, or mental illness. In essence, we have difficulty being empathic with those who are different from us. Thus we cannot assume that those who make societal decisions are indeed empathic.

As our society has become increasingly bureaucratic, people are distanced from the decisions that most affect them.[6] Because we often rely on others to represent us and our concerns, to the degree that we are different from those who represent us, we cannot be assured that they represent us empathically—and therefore, adequately. Further, in bureaucratic systems, empathic responses diminish as the responsibility for decisions becomes more routinized and impersonal. It becomes even more difficult to trust that those with power can empathize with the increasing diversity of people and issues that confront them.

Just as empathy is important to individual relationships, the expression of empathy is also crucial for societal relations, in the institutions and policies of that society. This "societal empathy" is seen in the ways that each society provides for those who are needy and sick and in society's willingness to embrace collective as well as individual misfortunes.

Societal empathy requires that those who make social policy decisions must be empathic with those for whom the decisions are made and with those who will be affected by these decisions. In health care this includes the caretakers as well as those who are cared for. In a society where those who make and influence social policy are generally of a different sex, race, or socio-economic background than those whom they are expected to represent, it may be particularly difficult for decision makers to be empathic with those who will be affected by their policies.

A Physician's Refrain

To underscore these points and to elucidate the complexity of the problem of societal empathy, I will describe the experience of "Jane Worthy, M.D.," a young woman whose story exemplifies the realities facing increasing numbers of young physicians in the United States today. Empathizing with her hopes, frustrations, and disappointments is essential to our understanding of her patients and our health care system.

Dr. Worthy is a thirty-two-year-old family practitioner, earning $70,000 a year, working in a group practice in a medium-sized city in a populous western state. She completed her residency two years ago, is a single parent, and has educational debts exceeding $80,000. She has taken a job in a large multispecialty group practice primarily because it will cover many of her overhead costs, including malpractice insurance. She had originally intended to return to practice in her hometown, where there is only one other physician, but she could not repay her loans and accrue the additional debt that would have been necessary if she were to open an independent practice. In addition, she could not have managed a demanding night and weekend call schedule without additional child care help, which she could not afford.

As individuals, we can empathize with the difficult choices she has had to make. There is, however, more to her story. We must also understand her position within a societal system that is empathic neither with her nor, perhaps, with us.

Recently, after her group practice contracted with a large managed care program, pressures began to mount for individual practitioners to see additional patients and to spend less time with each of those enrolled in the program. Limits were placed on requests for certain consultations and laboratory procedures. In addition, financial incentives were offered to those physicians who complied and thereby saved money for the practice. Individual physicians began to have less control over their schedules and their patients. Unless a new patient made a strong case with the receptionist/"gatekeeper" for direct physician intervention, the patient was assigned to see a nurse practitioner or physician's assistant for a brief evaluative session. Even long-standing patients were limited in their appointment times and contact with their physicians.

These changes increased Dr. Worthy's sense of isolation from her patients. Although she still delights in seeing them and their families and feels that she can make a difference in their lives, she is not certain that the future will permit her even this small reward. She is also growing more troubled by the "business" of medicine, as she finds herself focusing more on the fiscal aspects of practice and volumes of paperwork. She feels that she is not doing the best job for her patients, and she hesitates when asked whether she would go into medicine again, or if she would want her daughter to go into medicine. She considers leaving medicine altogether or changing specialties, although neither choice is desirable or realistic.

Even more distressing to her is the growing public negativism toward physicians: the suspicion, the anger, and the mistrust. This intensifies her anxiety about missing a diagnosis, making a mistake, or being sued. She feels especially vulnerable because there is less backup and support from colleagues, nurses, and the laboratory than existed a year ago. She is saddened by the lack of empathy for physicians. At the same time, she worries about the personal dangers of practicing medicine. She is concerned about the risks of physical assault or of contracting hepatitis, tuberculosis, or AIDS.

She is also troubled because, despite the need for physicians in family practice and primary care, the number of medical students choosing these specialties continues to be low.[7] By the early 1990s less than 20 percent of medical students indicated that they had "generalist" career preferences. Despite the widespread agreement about the need, there are insufficient incentives or supports to make it possible for those in debt to repay loans and to look forward to a style of life that would be less pressured. She knows that the choice of a higher-paying specialty would have helped her to pay off her debts more rapidly and to improve the quality of her life. If (as she predicts) specialty choices will increasingly become subject to economic constraints or even arbitrary limits on numbers of applicants, she is concerned that physicians will lose motivation and commitment.

Dr. Worthy is not optimistic about her future or about the future of health care in the United States. She, like many Americans, worries about deteriorating quality and lack of access to care as well as spiraling costs. Her perspective, however, is different from what we hear daily. She is not unempathic, she does care, and she is not greedy, selfish, or dishonest. How can we reconcile her concerns with the public's suspicions and with the overwhelming economic pressures? Can we become mutually empathic?

Medicine in Changing Times: Patients and Providers

Dr. Worthy's story depicts the experience of those working in a "system" that has undergone many changes in recent years. The potential for growing detachment and mistrust in both doctors and patients is evident. A contractual, business relationship threatens to take the place of the covenantal one held as our model in the past.[8] Although in practice this ideal was far from perfect, giving it up has had a profound effect on those providing care as well as on patients. Dr. Worthy's experience makes concrete what we have seen, that "trends toward entrepreneurship and organizational dependence are changing the structure of accountability within which physicians operate. Pressures on the physician to consider interests other than the patient's are increasing. Qualitative financial and organizational changes are taking place that may affect whether physicians will behave as if responsible first and foremost to meeting the needs of their patients."[9]

If we want to continue to embrace the spirit of beneficence and to value the relationship between care givers and patients, we must identify and alter practices that potentially undermine that relationship. Such practices distance physicians from their patients and put physicians in roles that are not necessarily in their patients' best interests. When physicians are expected to limit patients' access to health care by acting as gatekeepers or guardians of society's resources, for instances, they are not primarily their patients' advocates.[10] Although from an economic point of view it may be appealing to ask that the physician assume the role of gatekeeper, when the physician becomes a double or triple agent, acting for the government, an insurance company, an employer, and presumably for the patient and family as well, the nature of trust in the physician-patient relationship becomes ambiguous.

It has been argued that because gate-keeping functions will be inevitable in the future, it would be better to have a knowledgeable and compassionate physician in that role than a detached or less involved bureaucrat.[11] This argument, while pragmatic and even possibly empathic, implies that medicine must accept a different set of ethical principles and priorities than it currently holds. It places the physician in a conflict between the needs of the individual patient and the needs of society. One can argue that ultimately society, to be both just and fair, must impose this problem on physicians. Justice and fairness are compatible, however, only if we can be empathic.

A Bush administration directive underscored this dilemma. It prohibited physicians who worked in facilities that were recipients of government family-planning funds from discussing the option of abortion with their pregnant patients. In mandating that the physician withhold information from the patient, a fundamental principle of medical ethics was violated and the physician-patient relationship was encroached upon. The physician was prevented from acting responsibly and empathically, in the patient's best interests; and the patient was prevented from obtaining the objective and accurate information necessary for her to make an informed decision. Judgment and decision-making authority were placed in the hands of people with no direct involvement with, and perhaps little empathy for, women confronted by an unwanted pregnancy.

In recent years, in part because of the concern that physicians were not sufficiently empathic, there have been increasing expectations on the part of patients that they be informed participants in medical decision making. The locus of decision making, however, as this example and Dr. Worthy's experience so well illustrate, has shifted away from the physician, patient, and family and is more often found in the hands of governments, insurance companies, or other bureaucracies.[12]

The advent of these increasingly complex bureaucracies has placed constraints on medical practice that reinforce the barriers between individual providers and patients. Many of these constraints threaten to disrupt further the continuity of care and the already fragile empathic connection between patients and those providing care. Rigid time restrictions on the length of visits, the use of gatekeepers and other screening approaches, and prior-approval requirements have been designed to limit costs by limiting access to providers. The omnipresent threat of legal action, reinforced by the emphasis on commercial values, has also increased the distance between patients and providers. These changes have contributed to the feeling on the part of both physicians and patients that there is little empathy built into the systems that govern health care. Physicians believe that they are viewed more as technicians performing an assigned task than as professionals with a primary commitment to their patients. Patients experience the bureaucratization of health care as a series of continuous obstacles to good and compassionate care.

These structural changes also signal an interesting shift in the locus of paternalism in health care. Many of the manifestations of paternalistic and authoritarian behavior observed in the past in the practices of individual physicians are less evident today. Paternalism, however, is more apparent in the health care "system" itself. As a bureaucracy, this system, like all bureaucracies, is less likely to be empathic with the needs of individuals, or to take account of differences among patients. As Kathy Ferguson indicates, "The requirements of depersonalization in bureaucratic relations mean that individuals are isolated from one another and meaningful social interaction is replaced by formal association. . . . Bureaucracy separates people from one another in their activities, and from themselves in their roles."[13]

Increasing distance and isolation in the health care system is particularly troublesome because of the nature of illness and the vulnerability associated with it. Because responses to illness are often at variance with a person's usual behavior, the patient's understanding, judgment, and ability to make decisions or to consent to treatment may be compromised by an illness. Patients rely on those caring for them to provide information, explanation, and compassion. Their decisions are influenced by trusting relationships with their care givers and by their belief that their care givers possess the knowledge and ability required to be informative and helpful.[14] A "system" cannot take the place of individuals engaged in mutually participatory, empathic relationships. It is not in the nature of bureaucracy to be empathic.

Mutual participation and trust "helps to distinguish the doctor-patient relationship from commercial relationships in which the ethic of caveat emptor applies."[15] As Eliot Freidson has stated, "Rightly or wrongly, necessarily or unnecessarily, human health care serves diffuse human needs for being comforted and cared for as much as if not more than it serves organic, technically defined needs. If the comfort of human interactions were removed from health care by mechanization and patients were treated as mere bodies in the course of such mechanization, medical care would no longer serve most of the needs of today's patients."[16]

The Health Care System: How Are Women Treated?

The increasing inequities in the health care system over the last few decades have important implications for health care in general and for women specifically, given that women in the United States are more likely than men to have limited access to health care resources. Women are more often uninsured or underinsured, and they will be more adversely affected by policies that further limit the availability of health care.[17]

In the early 1970s many thought that if there were more women physicians, the authoritarian and hierarchical male-dominated model of medicine would give way to a more egalitarian one. This new model, it was assumed, would respond more empathically to women's concerns.[18] In retrospect, it appears that these expectations represented the victory of optimism over experience. The relative absence of women physicians, and women generally, from policymaking positions has minimized their ability to change the traditional authoritarian model. Currently it is the "system" rather than the individual physician that occupies the pivotal paternalistic position, as Dr. Worthy's story illustrates.

Our society has been portrayed as "gendered," that is, characterized by a "deeply entrenched institutionalization of sexual difference"[19] that pervades roles, policies, and attitudes, often without our conscious awareness or rational justification. In a gendered society, where those who dominate are expected to represent the whole, it may be difficult for men and women to be truly empathic with each other.

Women have increasingly been concerned over the lack of response on the part of government and the medical community to their health problems. Evidence is accumulating that there is a disparity both in research and in resource allocation that cannot be explained merely by happenstance. The "epidemic" of breast cancer in the United States, for example, did not initially generate the same kind of response with regard to research or funding as have other less prevalent diseases that primarily affected men.[20]

The failure to include female subjects in many research protocols, even in studies where sex differences might be expected to produce different outcomes, such as those involving medication doses, illustrates the point. The reasons given for these omissions included the objection that women would increase the cost and complexity of research because of the greater number of variables to take into account, such as menstrual cycles and pregnancy. Paradoxically, it also has been suggested that because men and women are so similar physiologically, the data from men could be extrapolated to women. Thus there would be no need to complicate the research further or increase costs by adding women to samples. The assumption that women and men are enough alike to extrapolate data obviously conflicts with the view that women can be excluded because their physiology is too different and complex.

Regardless of how we interpret these rationales, the result has been a startling lack of research on disorders that predominantly or substantially affect women. Although coronary artery disease occurs with greater frequency in men, for example, it is the leading cause of death in women. The paucity of data about women with this disease led the public, and even physicians, to conclude erroneously that women were at low risk. Consequently, this disease has been inadequately diagnosed and treated in women.[21]

A requirement that both male and female subjects be included in study designs, unless there is a specific reason not to do so, is an important step in improving our scientific integrity and redressing existing inequities.[22] The research discrepancy might also be mitigated by adding more women to the pool of researchers. Because researchers are most creative when they are working in areas that most engage them, at least some women investigators might find the study of women's health more challenging and rewarding.

As I have suggested, sex-related biases appear to influence recommendations for treatment as well as for research. Examination of the availability of organ transplants and bypass surgery reveals incongruities in criteria for the choice of suitable patients. Women and patients from minority populations are less frequently offered these options, without adequate medical justification.[23] Documentation of sex bias in medical care and in research has, in fact, led to the creation of an Office of Research on Women's Health in the National Institutes of Health.[24]

These issues raise important questions about the role of empathy in the delegation of decision-making authority. We have assumed that an empathic society can maintain objectivity while balancing the needs and wishes of those who are not directly represented. The examples I have given reinforce doubt that those in positions of power and influence have been as empathic to women as we hoped they would be. Skepticism has been increased by recent public experiences revealing how widely perceptions can differ about what constitutes violent assault, sexual harassment, or rape—for example, the Tailhook and Anita Hill–Clarence Thomas controversies.

The debate over the prohibition of the development or use of the abortifacient RU486 during the Reagan and Bush administrations also raised concerns about society's empathy for women. The limits placed on the production and availability of RU486 were based on the values and beliefs of those with decision-making authority at the time, without much empathy for the women who would potentially be affected. We can speculate about whether emphasizing the other possible uses of the drug, including the treatment of some types of breast cancer, brain tumors, Cushing's syndrome, and endometriosis, would have shifted the focus from the abortifacient properties of RU486; perhaps controlling its use for these purposes would have been less important to those seeking to prohibit it.

The lack of empathy and the paternalism represented in RU486 policy prior to 1994 are also demonstrated in the controversy over banning the use of fetal tissue for research. One of the central reasons given for this ban was the belief that more women would seek abortions if they felt there was such a justification for ending a pregnancy, or that "good" use could be made of the products of conception. This undocumented paternalistic belief implies that women cannot and should not make certain decisions, especially those with societal as well as individual implications.[25] The results may also be devastating to those with diseases such as Parkinsonism and diabetes, where there is promising research on the benefits of fetal tissue transplants.

The unique characteristics of women's reproductive role require special consideration because decisions about childbearing, contraception, abortion, sterilization, and reproductive surgery have profound societal consequences.[26] Women have often not participated in these decisions or consented to these procedures. Whether contraception or abortion is legal or funded can determine whether a woman can realistically make certain life choices. Unfortunately, women's interests are often not represented in these policy deliberations.[27]

The problem of empathy in societal decisions is also illustrated when a Caesarean section is recommended to protect a fetus, and the pregnant woman refuses. In most of these cases courts have dictated that the procedure be performed, holding the fetal right to life as superseding the woman's right to make a decision about the integrity and control of her body. More recently, however, this position has been rejected and the right of the pregnant woman to make the decision has been affirmed. The reasoning, in one case, stemmed from a decision that a man did not have to take the risk required to donate a kidney to his child.[28]

A British ethicist noted that the issue of forced Caesarean section most often arises in cases involving poor or foreign women, or women whose religious beliefs differ from those of the physician. This suggests that the cultural or socioeconomic dissimilarity between doctor and patient may have been a factor in the recommendation.[29] It also lends support to the view that it is difficult to be empathic with those who are different.

A related controversy involves whether failure to consent to the treatment of an in-utero fetus constitutes fetal abuse. Conceptualizing the problem in this way implies that the fetus and the pregnant woman are equal persons with equal rights, and that the pregnant woman has committed a crime—abuse—against another person, a fetus. A distinction between a pregnant woman and her fetus has been made by the American Medical Association. It holds that a woman cannot be coerced to accept a treatment solely to benefit her fetus, and that it is the physician's ethical duty to be noncoercive and to accept that he/she can act only with the informed consent of the patient.[30] This decision represents a statement of rights and respect, and perhaps also illustrates empathy for the pregnant woman.

An Experiment in Priority Setting: Cost, Benefit, and Empathy

I argue against unremitting adherence to strictly "objective," predetermined criteria in health policy. On the contrary, health policy decisions must be flexible enough to allow for an empathic approach to individual cases that cannot be pressed into a Procrustean bed of objectivity.

The emphasis on developing objective criteria is problematic, because inevitably the results are more subjective than is implied by the apparently objective conclusions that are reached. Further, the criteria do not necessarily arise from empathic or compassionate considerations, nor do they deal adequately with special circumstances or contingencies, such as age, sex, or severity of illness. For example, a decision might be made, as was the case in Oregon in the 1980s, to stop funding transplant surgery. Does this decision apply to all transplants, including those that are relatively inexpensive or of proven efficacy? What happens when the technology is improved, the costs decrease, and the procedure is more widely accepted? Are there special circumstances or considerations that might mitigate the rule? How should we differentiate the case of a two-year-old who needs a bone marrow transplant from the eighty-year-old who needs a cardiac transplant? When resources are limited, would other circumstances affect priority scores, such as favoring the person who has responsibility for the care of young children? These are not new questions; they have been agonized over in intensive care units and emergency rooms for decades, but they have rarely been the subject of open public policy discussion or debate.

A recent and revolutionary attempt to define and apply ostensibly objective standards to the allocation of resources for health care was undertaken by the state of Oregon.[31] In an effort to consider alternative approaches to providing health care for the poor, a complex algorithm was generated to develop and rate priorities for treatment. It took account of benefit to the patient by making a subjective assessment of quality of life improvement over time. I will briefly summarize the plan and some of the pros and cons of its approach, focusing on aspects of this effort that relate to societal empathy.

At the time of the first public presentation of the Oregon plan, more than seven hundred services were ranked by order of priority based on an estimate of need for service and efficacy of intervention. A cutoff for services was determined, based on estimated state fiscal resources. The list then defined the services to be provided. Those that fell below the cutoff figure were not funded. They would not be available to patients who depended on the state to finance their health care.

This process resulted in coverage for some services that had not previously been covered, and in the removal of coverage for others that previously had been covered. Ostensibly, it made sense to cover more serious conditions that were deemed medically necessary. For instance, hospice care was covered, but bursitis, diaper rash, and the common cold were not.[32] But because severity of illness and special circumstances were not addressed, a common cold in an eighty-year-old widow with cardiac disease who lived alone was not treated differently from the same illness in a healthy college student. Despite the potential difference in seriousness, neither patient would be covered. Likewise, a fifteen-year-old single mother might not learn how to care for her infant's diaper rash and prevent more serious consequences, because that condition was not covered in the plan.

The priority scores for four treatments in the list originally provided by the Oregon Health Services Commission illustrate another conceptual problem with that approach. The first pass in the process of assigning priority scores produced a list that rated tooth capping at 371, surgery for ectopic pregnancy at 372, splints for temporomandibular joint disorder at 376, and appendectomy at 377.[33] That two of these procedures are life-saving with a virtually 100 percent chance of recovery, and the others by comparison are elective, did not translate into what could be considered a rational outcome.

These counterintuitive results led to a reconsideration of the proposed plan. In part this occurred because it was argued that the initial assignment of priority scores objectified health care in a way that did not take account of human suffering or of the impact of denying life-saving procedures. That the list "seemed to favor minor treatments over lifesaving ones . . . reflects a fundamental and irreconcilable conflict between cost-effectiveness analysis and the powerful human proclivity to rescue endangered life."[34]

Obviously, one cannot compare tooth capping with surgery for an ectopic pregnancy, either for the individual or for society at large, unless one takes a strict (and perhaps skewed) utilitarian approach. The consultants also estimated that "70 percent of patients with ectopic pregnancy would die if not operated on."[35] Suppose that a woman with an ectopic pregnancy is among the 70 percent who die, and that she would leave six children motherless. How are the ramifications of her death accounted for in the priority-setting process? One does not, of course, need such a dramatic or obvious example to question the ethical problems raised by rationing health care generally, or using this plan specifically.

Proponents of the Oregon plan emphasize that it expands access to care by providing universal coverage; it focuses on clinical effectiveness and not primarily on costs; and it tackles the difficult and controversial problem of defining what constitutes "basic" care. It also involves considerable "consumer" input. Although societal empathy would support—indeed, would require—consumer input in the process of priority setting, it was not clear how representative the consumer groups were; how they were chosen; what preparation, information, and instructions they were given; or how their input was collected and used.

The Oregon system was designed to redistribute existing resources so that taxes need not increase to support the growing health care expenses of the poor; access to private health insurance benefits would be available to those who so chose. Those opposed to the plan feel that because it is only for people on public assistance, it rations care primarily for the poor; those who are more affluent are less affected. Critics also suggest that in eliminating coverage for those illnesses that were judged to be of lower priority, the plan could change what is considered "basic" annually, as the state budget changed. In addition, critics point out that issues of severity of illness and prevention are not sufficiently addressed.

Insofar as "rationing is far easier to accept as an abstract necessity than for an identified individual,"[36] approaches that are societally empathic—that confront us with the reality of individuals whose lives and well-being are affected—must be utilized. For example, critics of the plan assert that the plan not only is burdensome for the poor but is specifically burdensome for poor women and children. Although others have refuted this claim, poor women and children do constitute 75 percent of the Medicaid recipients who would be affected by the plan.[37] This is the case not only in Oregon but in the United States generally. Women are far more likely to receive health care coverage from public sources, and men, from private sources.[38] Further, because the majority of the elderly are women, and the elderly are the greatest consumers of health care, any program designed to dispense public funding for health care is more likely to affect women disproportionately.[39]

The problem of developing plans that are empathetic and humane remains a major challenge. "No sector of the health care system appears to be uniquely compassionate and caring . . . the heart of the problem created by the objectification of medical care is not the risk to such amenities as common courtesy, but the danger that the impersonal criteria that are set for categories of patients will be inappropriately applied to individual patients and that care will be strictly limited to that which has been contracted for."[40]

The effort that went into development of the Oregon plan was extraordinary and unique, albeit flawed. Imperfection should not lead to a global rejection of these efforts, but it does argue for ongoing exploration and evaluation of proposed alternative models and a commitment to remaining cognizant of the human dimension and the need for societal empathy.

The last few decades have brought changes in traditionally held views of the responsibilities, obligations, and relationships between health care providers and patients. It is no longer clear who is the patient's advocate. The increasing complexity and cost of medical technology, coupled with limited resources to provide care for all those who need or want it, have expanded the scope of the health policy discussion to include issues not previously considered. Decision making in medicine has always been substantially influenced by competing priorities, but policies regarding who should make decisions and what the priorities should be must be reexamined in a contemporary context. Choices that enable one to be empathetic and to preserve personal moral accountability in a pluralistic society are difficult to make.

The health policy debate has been pushed into the economic arena, and patient concerns and participation have generally been subsumed by these pressures. "More and more the services received by patients are not the result of a decision of a single person who is accountable to the patient but are instead the product of negotiations between providers and payers. The interests of patients will not be served if patient care decisions are excessively influenced by payer-created economic incentives or determinations of appropriateness."[41]

In short, the role of the individual voice in health policy decisions is increasingly threatened by growing bureaucratization. Empathy is essential to providing good health care; societal empathy is a prerequisite for ethical and compassionate health policy. As a society, we must develop the structures that promote these values. We must hear those, like Jane Worthy, who recognize that the danger in losing our empathy is losing our humanity.

Notes

This paper was prepared while the author was a Fellow at the Center for Advanced Study in the Behavioral Sciences. She is grateful for the financial support provided by the John D. and Catherine T. MacArthur Foundation.

1. Arnold H. Modell, *Other Times, Other Realities: Toward a Theory of Psychoanalytic Treatment* (Cambridge, Mass.: Harvard University Press, 1990).

2. Heinz Kohut, "The Psychoanalyst in the Community of Scholars," in *The Search for the Self: Selected Writings of Heinz Kohut*, vol. 2, ed. Paul Ornstein, (New York: International Universities Press, 1978), 685–724.

3. Eric J. Cassell, "Recognizing Suffering," *Hastings Center Report* 21:3 (May–June 1991):24–31.

4. Ibid., 24.

5. Alfred Margulies, *The Empathic Imagination* (New York: W. W. Norton and Co., 1989).

6. Kathy Ferguson, *The Feminist Case against Bureaucracy* (Philadelphia: Temple University Press, 1984).

7. David A. Kindig, James M. Cultice, and Fitzhugh Mullan, "The Elusive Generalist Physician," *Journal of the American Medical Association* 270:9 (September 1, 1993):1069–1073.

8. E. Pellegrino and D. Thomasma, *For the Patient's Good* (New York: Oxford University Press, 1988).

9. Bradford H. Gray, *The Profit Motive and Patient Care* (Cambridge, Mass.: Harvard University Press, 1991), 172.

10. Pellegrino and Thomasma, *For the Patient's Good*; Carol C. Nadelson, "Presidential Address—Health Care Directions: Who Cares for Patients?" *American Journal of Psychiatry* 143 (1986):949–955.

11. Howard Brody, *The Healer's Power* (New Haven: Yale University Press, 1992).

12. Carol C. Nadelson, "Emerging Issues in Medical Ethics," *British Journal of Psychiatry* 158 (Supp. 10, 1991):9–16.

13. Ferguson, *The Feminist Case*, 13.

14. Carol C. Nadelson and Malkah T. Notman, "Adaptation to Stress in Physicians," *Becoming a Physician*, ed. E. Shapiro and L. Lowenstein (Cambridge, Mass.: Ballinger, 1979), 201–216.

15. Gray, *The Profit Motive*, 169.

16. Eliot Freidson, *Doctoring Together* (New York: Elsevier, 1975), 326.

17. U.S. National Institutes of Health, *Report: U.S. National Institutes of Health*, September 10, 1990; Nancy S. Jecker, "Age-Based Rationing and Women," *Journal of the American Medical Association* 266:21 (1991):3012–3015.

18. Nadelson and Notman, "Adaptation to Stress."

19. Susan Moller Okin, *Justice, Gender, and the Family* (New York: Basic Books, 1989).

20. U.S. National Institutes of Health, *Report: U.S. National Institutes*.

21. John Z. Ayanian and Arnold M. Epstein, "Differences in the Use of Procedures between Women and Men Hospitalized for Coronary Heart

Disease," *New England Journal of Medicine* 325:4 (July 25, 1991):221–230; Richard M. Steingart, Milton Packer, Peggy Hamm, Mary E. Coglianese et al., "Sex Differences in the Management of Coronary Artery Disease," *New England Journal of Medicine* 325:4 (July 25, 1991):226–230.

22. U.S. National Institutes of Health, *Report: U.S. National Institutes.*

23. L. Abraham, "Transplants Available for Young, White, Wealthy Men," *American Medical News* (January 7, 1991); U.S. National Institutes of Health, *Report: U.S. National Institutes.*

24. U.S. National Institutes of Health, *Report: U.S. National Institutes*; J. Palca, "Women Left Out at NIH," *Science* 148 (1990):1601–1602.

25. "Doctors Plan to Review Fetal Tissue Research," *Boston Globe* (January 8, 1991); P. J. Hilts, "Groups Set Up Panel on Use of Fetal Tissue," *New York Times* (January 8, 1991).

26. Carol C. Nadelson and Malkah T. Notman, "Emotional Aspects of the Symptoms, Functions and Disorders of Women," *Psychiatric Medicine,* ed. G. Usdin (New York: Brunner/Mazel, 1979).

27. Nadelson, "Emerging Issues."

28. Henry Shenkin, *Medical Ethics: Evolution, Rights, and the Physician* (Dordrecht: Kluwer Academic, 1991).

29. Ibid.

30. American Medical Association, "Sexual Misconduct in the Practice of Medicine," report of the Council on Ethical and Judicial Affairs of the AMA., presented to and passed by the House of Delegates in Miami, Miami, Fla., December 19, 1990.

31. David M. Eddy, "Oregon's Plan: Did Cost-Effectiveness Analysis Fail?" *Journal of the American Medical Association* 266:15 (October 16, 1991):2135–2141.

32. David M. Eddy, "Oregon's Plan: Should It Be Approved?" *Journal of the American Medical Association* 266:17 (November 6, 1991):2439–2445.

33. David C. Hadorn, "Setting Health Care Priorities in Oregon: Cost-Effectiveness Meets the Rule of Rescue," *Journal of the American Medical Association* 265:17 (1991):2218–2225.

34. Ibid.

35. Ibid.

36. Charles J. Dougherty, "Setting Health Care Priorities: Oregon's Next Steps," *Hastings Center Report* 21:3 (May–June 1991):1–10.

37. Norman Daniels, "Is the Oregon Rationing Plan Fair?" *Journal of the American Medical Association* 265:17 (May 1, 1991):2232–2235.

38. Charlotte F. Muller, *Health Care and Gender* (New York: Russell Sage Foundation, 1990).

39. A trial of a revised version of the plan is currently being undertaken in Oregon, but its final form is undetermined at the time of this writing.

40. Gray, *The Profit Motive,* 327.

41. Ibid., 324.

RITA CHARON, MICHELE G. GREENE,
AND RONALD ADELMAN

Women Readers, Women Doctors

A Feminist Reader-Response Theory for Medicine

The love of our neighbor in all its fullness simply means being able to say to him, "What are you going through?"

Simone Weil, *Waiting for God*

The relationship between a patient and a doctor is the medium in which medical care occurs, fundamentally influencing the effectiveness of individual health care.[1] In attempts to improve the dividends of medical care, researchers have studied the doctor-patient relationship to learn what contributes to clinical effectiveness. Patient characteristics such as age, gender, and preparedness to ask questions and physician characteristics such as gender, specialty, and training in interviewing skills have all been shown to influence the process and outcome of the medical interaction.[2]

The study of medical interactions, however, has been hampered by the lack of explanatory models robust enough to capture the complexity of doctor-patient work. Instead, medical interactions conventionally are interpreted as sets of random, unifunctional behaviors bent toward instrumental goals rather than as singular interpersonal events rich in ambiguity and marked by mutual responsiveness.[3] Until models sufficiently complex are applied to medical interactions, studies of these interactions will result in misleading or unhelpful findings.

We have been engaged in research studies of doctor-patient interactions for almost a decade. Initially interested in the special features of geriatric medicine, we audiotape-recorded interviews between doctors and their elderly patients and examined these taped conversations with the use of a linguistic analytic instrument of our design to document the presence of ageism in the clinical encounter. We have since examined other aspects of the medical interaction, including the influence of the patient's and physician's gender on the process and content of the medical interview.[4] To explore the influence of the doctor's gender on events in the medical interview, we studied sixty medical interviews between doctors and their patients at routine medical follow-up visits, comparing the interviews of women internists with those of men internists seeing patients from the same population in the same setting. Before reporting on the methods used to study the interactions and the differences documented between the interviews of women doctors and those of men doctors, it may be helpful to outline the conceptual framework we adopted in developing the hypotheses and interpreting the findings.

A Narrative Model of Medical Interactions

One model that may capture some of the complexity of the doctor-patient interaction is a narrative model. Including such forms as novels, newspaper stories, jokes, history, and scripture, narratives tell stories by arranging events in a temporally meaningful order, allowing a plot to unfold, and establishing a signifying relationship between teller and listener. Doctors and patients, this model suggests, are engaged in complex interpretive activities that are language-based, that include cognitive and affective components, and that combine objective factual deliberations with subjective interpersonal engagement. The aim of the medical narrative enterprise is, like that of any narrative, the search for meaning within temporally complex and semiotically chaotic texts and events. Because medical events are human events and because, as Jerome Bruner comments, "we organize our experience and our memory of human happenings mainly in the form of narrative—stories, excuses, myths, reasons for doing and not doing, and so on," adopting a narrative framework to investigate medical interactions may clarify their processes and outcomes.[5] The events of illness are embedded in the seamless continuous events of the patient's life, and therefore comprehensive patient care ideally requires that doctors fully understand their patients' narratives of illness in all their complexities—the reports of symptoms as well as the account of attendant emotional states, familial concerns, attributions of significance and cause of the symptoms, and ramifications of illness and care. To hear such concerns, doctors must attend not only to explicit statements but to the unsaid implications, the nonverbal communications, and the affective "envelope" as well as to the objective findings of physical examination and laboratory testing. Narrative understandings of the practice of and the teaching of medicine may help doctors to achieve these goals of care.[6]

A narrative model further suggests that, in performing diagnostic and therapeutic work, doctors process information and make decisions using narrative methods. To interpret the narrative of a sick patient, a doctor needs to establish the sequence of events, to examine the relationship between events and the motivations and responses of the people involved, to assert causal connections among events, and to contextualize the events within the relevant frames. Furthermore, doctors need to recognize the multiple perspectives of an illness, to acknowledge their own responses to patients, and to reconcile the diverse and oftentimes contradictory messages obtained about an illness. The doctor's task, one might say, is to offer a medical interpretation that incorporates and explains the patient's story and leads to useful action.[7]

Finally, doctors and patients join in the hard work of choosing the relevant facts and seeking coherence in a chaotic combination of illness events, life events, physical sensations, laboratory findings, responses to treatment, and emotions of all concerned. Although doctor and patient have fundamentally different tasks to do within the illness, they join in tolerating uncertainty, taking risks, and accepting the inevitable. Whether dealing with a reversible, chronic, or terminal illness, doctor and patient each—if the relationship is an effective one—influence the course of events and recognize the nature of and the meaning of the events befalling them.

The Act of Reading

Among the aspects of the doctor's work clarified by a narrative model of medicine are recognition of the patient's problem, attentiveness to the patient's narrative, constructing a coherent interpretation of findings, and hearing the patient to the end. These skills can be grouped conceptually as acts of reading, for these acts of recognition, interpretation, and perspectival knowledge bring the doctor in contact with a patient's story in the way that a novel or short story transports a reader into the narrative world of the teller. Although the clinical situation differs markedly from the reading situation, both are instances of narrative discourse, described by Barbara Herrnstein Smith as "verbal acts consisting of *someone telling someone else that something happened,*" and can be inspected using similar conceptual tools.[8]

When doctors diagnose and treat patients, they rely on the skills that readers use to achieve appropriate distance and engagement, to combine objective and subjective knowledge into a fruitful personal knowledge, to recognize their own not insignificant contribution to the meanings of stories, and to enter into narrative worlds.[9] Readers achieve the meanings of a text by identifying the genre of a work and accepting its conventions, contextualizing it within its time period and tradition, critically examining its form and diction, mentally cohering the text's images and events and language while responding emotionally to the plot and the characters, associating to personal memories, becoming engaged in the struggles of the characters, and being personally affected by the outcome. Calling reading an "astonishing process . . . in [which] we are able to experience things that no longer exist and to understand things that are totally unfamiliar to us," Wolfgang Iser describes a balancing act in which the reader "oscillates between involvement in and observation of those illusions; he opens himself to the unfamiliar world without being imprisoned in it. . . . A literary text must therefore be conceived in such a way that it will engage the reader's imagination in the task of working things out for himself, for reading is only a pleasure when it is active and creative."[10]

Because theoreticians of reading, beginning with Aristotle, have developed a complex and nuanced understanding of the process that occurs between reader and text, medicine might do well to borrow that which applies to its own interactional enterprise in the search for robust new conceptual models for understanding itself.[11] The doctor, understood within a narrative framework, is "reading" the texts of the patient—the oral tale, the affective presence, the hospital chart, the physical findings, the laboratory tracings and images—hoping to achieve the clinical equivalent of the aesthetic satisfaction of reading. The doctor hopes, that is, to fashion a coherent interpretation of contradictory messages by using all his or her "active and creative" faculties of perception, cognition, and affective response to reach a proper diagnosis and recommend helpful treatment.

How can this parallel between medical work and reading help to investigate differences between women doctors and men doctors? Contemporary feminist and post-structuralist literary critics have been studying the gendered aspects of reading and writing, asserting that reading and writing are activities that implicate corporeal and culturally learned gender identity. Feminist critics have examined ways in which women read differently from men: women and men predictably achieve different interpretations of the same texts employing different reading strategies in so doing. Factors that make women readers different from men readers may be among the factors that make women doctors different from men doctors; gender issues in reading then may illuminate gender issues in medicine.

Feminist Theories of Reading

One of the early tasks embraced by feminist literary critics was the description of the woman reading. Women readers, it was asserted, read differently from men, switching gender affiliation to understand a story by or about men and "filling in the blanks" in reading texts written by or about women. Because most texts in the traditional literary canon are written by and about men, women readers must cross-identify in reading a great deal more than must men, causing women readers to divide themselves to adopt the male perspective.[12] An early investigator of the gendered aspects of reading, Annette Kolodny, suggested that "whether we speak of poets and critics 'reading' texts or writers 'reading' (and thereby recording for us) the world, we are calling attention to interpretive strategies that are learned, historically determined, and thereby necessarily gender-inflected."[13] Differentiating itself from a concurrent literary scholarship that emphasizes the "new sciences of the text . . . strenuous, rigorous, impersonal, and virile" and aims to achieve replicable solutions to textual problems, "the task of feminist critics is to find a new language, a new way of reading that can integrate our intelligence and our experience, our reason and our suffering, our skepticism and our vision. This enterprise should not be confined to women."[14]

A hallmark of feminist criticism is the attention to the silent, the hidden, and the subterranean features of the novels of women authors. In their authoritative treatment of nineteenth-century women authors, Sandra Gilbert and Susan Gubar describe women's works as "palimpsestic, works whose surface designs conceal or obscure deeper, less accessible (and less socially acceptable) levels of meaning."[15] The task of reading such works calls forth a level of participation and attentiveness not always required and achieved only by readers committed to understanding all levels of meaning contained within them. The attentive reader uses the imagination and the empathy that is needed by the attentive physician leaning toward the patient, man or woman, who is burdened with a story whose inner meaning often remains hidden from the teller until a skillful hearing reveals it. The patient—who may feel powerless in front of a medical system of authority, who may feel helpless against physical symptoms and emotional fears, who may be hiding aspects of the meaning of illness events—may indeed, like the woman author, be telling a muted story concealed within a dominant biomedical and socially acceptable story. A leading figure in French feminist criticism, Hélène Cixous, describes the woman reader in terms that may also be applied to the ideal care giver, "She who observes with a gaze that recognizes, studies, respects, doesn't seize or make marks, but attentively, with a gentle stubbornness, contemplates and reads, caresses, bathes, makes the other radiant."[16]

Related to the way that women's working groups may choose

collaborative over competitive styles or that young girls may understand moral questions relationally and contextually rather than through
application of abstract principles, women readers have been found to
approach texts using their personal experiences more openly and falling back less frequently than men on abstract formulations of rules of
interpretation.[17] In an essay on Emily Dickinson, the poet and critic
Adrienne Rich writes, "For years I have been not so much envisioning
Emily Dickinson as trying to visit, to enter her mind, through her poems and letters, and through my own intimations of what it could have
meant to be [her]."[18] Here is a reader using her imagination to re-create
the world and inner reality of her author, not inventing her from afar
but nearing and visiting, accepting her works on her own ground. In a
commentary on Rich's essay, Patricinio Schweickart notes Rich's "tendency to construe the text not as an object, but as the manifestation of
the subjectivity of the absent author—the 'voice' of another woman."[19]
Is this quality peculiar to Adrienne Rich as a critic or does her gender
influence her approach to a poem?

Many feminists answer that question with a resounding assertion
that the woman reader—by virtue of having been a daughter and not a
son, by virtue of her experience in the nondominant sphere of social
life, by virtue of her historical and familial role as care giver and
nurturer, by virtue of the patriarchial structures that disdain women's
experiences and isolate power among men—tenders toward her texts
more attentiveness and recognition than does the man reader.[20] Without committing epistemic leaps of confidence in female authority and
without subscribing to a biological essentialism, one can carefully examine women's characteristic moves toward finding meaning in texts
by looking clearly at the actual experiences of women and men readers. Because of the parallels between reading and doctoring, such understanding of women readers' acts may clarify women doctors'
characteristic moves toward finding meaning with their patients.

In an attempt to document gendered reading in nonprofessional readers, Elizabeth Flynn studied a large group of college students, comparing male students' interpretations of stories with female students'
interpretations. Flynn assigned short stories by James Joyce, Ernest
Hemingway, and Virginia Woolf to undergraduate students and collected their written narrative responses. Women and men readers differed consistently in the extent to which they resisted engagement with
the text, judged it, and were able to resolve its emotional tensions. Men
readers fell victim more often than women to "extremes of rejection or
identification, responses which interfered with their understanding of
the story," while women readers demonstrated more "discernment of

the limitations of the characters" and incorporated all details of the story's setting, images, and diction to arrive at critical readings.[21] Flynn concludes that women seem more able than men to achieve a balance between critical distance from a text and involvement with it, thereby evaluating the events and characters with empathic judgment that recognizes the meaningfulness of the stories, whereas men were more likely to react to stories by either turning away from them or attempting to dominate or control them.

What can explain this gender asymmetry? David Bleich reports on a similar experiment among graduate students in a comparative literature course. Aware that he was looking for "contingent regularity" rather than strict biological districting, he collected responses from male and female students and searched for patterns of difference in their reading acts. Bleich and his assistants found gender differences in the students' responses to prose fiction but not to lyrical poetry. He concludes that the differences, related to the narrative contract found in fiction and not in poetry, involved men's and women's different abilities to perceive "the 'voice' in the literature. . . . In the narrative, men perceived a strong narrative voice, but women experienced the narrative as a 'world,' without a particularly strong sense that this world was narrated into existence. . . . [W]omen *enter* the world of the novel, take it as something 'there' for that purpose; men *see* the novel as a result of someone's action and construe its meaning or logic in those terms."[22] Bleich notes that women students were more able to identify the emotional tensions in a story, the men restricting themselves to abstracting the facts of the case and not grasping the emotional undercurrents: "The women 'become' the tellers of the tales that they are reading. . . . Neither the teller nor the tale is radically other for the women" whereas the men "draw boundaries much more decisively. . . . The novels were more self-consciously *appropriated* by the men than by the women."[23]

Relying on psychoanalytic theories of language acquisition and gender differences in individuating from the mother, Bleich suggests that women readers are less impelled to remove themselves from narrating language. Because girls differentiate themselves less drastically from the "mother tongue" than do boys, who in gender identification must constitute themselves as other than the first speaker in their consciousness (the mother), women readers are better equipped to enter texts without experiencing threats to their identity, whereas men readers remain at a greater distance from language-mediated experience.

Emerging findings in object-relations psychology concerning the experiences of preoedipal daughters and sons (at least in middle-class, predominantly white, Western culture) may supply explanations of these differences in language acquisition. Says Nancy Chodorow, "Preoedipal experiences of girls and boys differ. . . . [M]others of daughters tend not to experience these infant daughters as separate from them in the same way as mothers of infant sons," these differences leading to developmental issues for women relating to "boundary confusion and a lack of sense of separateness from the world" for the girls but not for the boys.[24] If we interpret this somewhat differently, Chodorow is giving a psychoanalytic foundation for Bleich's findings of gendered reading: the women engaged more successfully with the voice of the other (the text), perhaps in part because of their freedom from boundary-marking, while the men, intent on distinguishing themselves from the voice of the text, were hampered from engaging with it by their need for boundaries. These gender differences may contribute to the empirical findings summarized by Flynn: a woman reader "learns from the experience without losing critical distance; reader and text interact with a degree of mutuality. . . . Self and other remain distinct and so create a kind of dialogue."[25]

Although research in gender differences in reading has just recently begun, it is clear that the field has identified concerns of fundamental importance. Jonathan Culler suggests that "to read as a woman" is a defining performance of a chosen and identifying role.[26] To read as a woman, then, may ultimately be approached as an explanatory framework in its own right, implying not biological essentialism but cultural commonalities—an articulation of the personal intimacy of interpreting narratives, of responding to language, and of making oneself available to comprehending an other.

Gender Influence in Medical Interviews: Content and Process

The feminist conceptual models of gendered reading can be applied to the results of a study of women doctors and men doctors talking with their patients: if women readers use characteristic practices in searching for meaning in texts, might women doctors use similar practices in understanding patients? We performed our study in a Northeast urban academic medical center, comparing the interactions of five women internists with the interactions of six men internists working in a medical out-patient department of a tertiary-care hospital caring for a predominantly elderly, minority, and poor patient population. The physician sample was randomly selected, and each physician in the sample was studied with both men and women patients. Sixty medical encounters were examined. We used the Geriatric Interaction Analysis instrument, a reliable and valid linguistic analytic system tailored to examining medical encounters, to analyze these audiotape-recorded visits.

Briefly, the Geriatric Interaction Analysis instrument permits coding of medical conversations directly from audiotapes. As a coder listens to a tape-recorded interview, he or she lists topics as they are raised in the conversation, noting whether the doctor or the patient raised the topic. The coder assesses the doctor's responsiveness to each topic by rating his or her performance of three interviewing behaviors—questioning, informing, and demonstrating support—on a four-point scale (comprehensive, sufficient, insufficient, or absent). Extensive coding rules guide coders' assessments; coders have routinely achieved about 80 percent agreement on inter-rater reliability testing.

Topics discussed during the medical visit are grouped into categories for statistical analysis, and the categories further aggregated into major content areas. In the study we report here, conversational categories were grouped into five major content areas—biomedical, psychosocial, personal habits, patient-physician relationship, and other. For example, categories such as work and leisure, family or significant other, bereavement, crime and victimization, and money and benefits are grouped in the psychosocial content area; categories such as alcohol use, sleep, sex, and drug use were grouped in the personal habits content area.

In addition to assessing the doctor's responsiveness in questioning, informing, and supportiveness, the Geriatric Interaction Analysis instrument also tracks such mutual behaviors as shared laughter and shared decision making. Global assessments are made at the end of the interactions for both patient and physician: coders use a five-point scale to rate patient characteristics of assertiveness, friendliness, relaxation, and expressiveness whereas physicians are rated on demonstrated levels of egalitarianism, patience, engagement, and respect. This interaction analysis system affords more contextualization than other available systems used in the medical setting. Rather than fragmenting doctor-patient conversations through tallies of isolated behaviors, as other methods do, this system emphasizes the responsive nature of the conversation. Consciously listening to the conversation many times from both the point of view of the patient and the physician, the coder achieves an interpretation of the meaning of the conversation.

Although this semiquantitative method does not replace close textual analysis of transcripts in linguistic study of conversations, it allows the investigator to aggregate findings across many interactions

and to test for broad influences of independent variables on the content
or the process of medical visits. We designed this study initially to test
the hypothesis that the age of the patient predicted specific behaviors
within the interview. The currently reported study was a secondary
analysis, testing hypotheses about the influence of the gender of the
physician on the process and content of the interview. Because coders
who studied the tapes were not aware of the study hypotheses, observer bias was limited.

Within the narrative conceptual framework grounded in feminist theories about the gendered activities of interpreting stories, attending to
affective and relational concerns, and entering narrative worlds, we
hypothesized that there would be several differences between women
and men doctors. We predicted that, in the aggregate: (1) women physicians would demonstrate more interest and engagement in life story
narratives told by their patients; (2) that women physicians would exercise less control over content and process of the visit than would
men; (3) that women physicians would, in view of a higher achievement of mutuality, provide more comprehensive information than
would men; (4) that women physicians would show a higher degree of
responsiveness to the patients than would men; and (5) that woman
physicians would spend more time with each patient and engage more
often in such mutual behaviors as shared laughter and joint decision
making than would men physicians. In broad strokes, these were the
behavioral and interactional correlates of a feminist theory of attentiveness, responsiveness, and narrative flexibility. In effect, the study hypothesized that the women physicians would differ from the men in
accomplishing the "reading" components of medical work and that the
women would repeat in medical work the gender differences demonstrated so far in studies of reading.

Results

We documented statistically significant differences between women and
men physicians in multiple dimensions of the interactions. Analyses of
variance were used to examine the effects of physician gender and
patient gender on selected aspects of the medical interview. With a few
exceptions, the patient's gender did not influence the findings of differences between men and women physicians.

What did the doctors and patients talk about, and did the gender of
the doctor influence the content of their conversation? Both men and
women patients raised significantly more medical topics with women
physicians than with men physicians ($p = .02$). Patients initiated dis-

cussion of personal habits (smoking, alcohol use, drug use, sex, sleep) significantly more often with women physicians than with men (p = .05); this area of discussion was influenced by patient gender, with men patients more likely to initiate discussion of personal habits with women physicians than with men physicians, and men patients altogether initiating more discussion of these topics than did women patients. Both men and women patients were significantly more likely to initiate discussion about psychosocial issues (family, work, money, emotional topics) with women physicians than with men physicians (p = .05). There was no statistical difference in the number of topics raised by women and men physicians.

Did women doctors differ from men doctors in their interviewing behaviors? Aggregating the interviewing behaviors of physicians in the areas of questioning, informing, and demonstrating support to patients through the course of the conversation, women physicians were significantly more responsive than were men physicians when patients (of either sex) initiated discussions on psychosocial topics (p = .03), though they were no different from men when discussing non-psychosocial topics. Women physicians were also more comprehensive in offering information to patients in discussing doctor-initiated psychosocial issues (p = .05) and were more supportive when patients raised psychosocial issues for discussion (p = .02).

Finally, did the interviews of women doctors differ from those of men doctors in global aspects of mutuality and overall assessments of doctor and patient characteristics? Women physicians spent more time with their patients than did men physicians, with an aggregated difference in visit time of 3 minutes and 51 seconds (p = .03). There was more likely to be shared laughter and shared decision making in visits with women physicians than with men physicians (p = .10 and p = .004).

The global assessments of physicians and patients differed according to physician gender. Women physicians were significantly more egalitarian (p < .001), more patient (p = .01), more engaged (p = .05), and more respectful (p = .009) than the men physicians. Patients were found to be more assertive with women physicians than with men physicians (p < .001); the other global assessments of patients did not differ with gender of physician.

All our hypotheses except hypothesis (2) were confirmed or partially confirmed by the findings. (1) Women physicians were more attentive, informative, and supportive to their patients when patients initiated discussion about life events, emotions, and relationships. (2) Women physicians were no different from men physicians, however, in the amount of control exerted in the visit, measured by the percentage of discussions that the doctor initiated. (3) Women physicians offered more comprehensive information to patients in the psychosocial content area. (4) Women physicians were more supportive of patients who raised issues of emotional or relational content. In addition, they were significantly more engaged, respectful, egalitarian, and patient than men physicians. (5) Finally, women physicians were more likely to engage in joint decision making and shared laughter with their patients, and they spent more time with their patients than did the men physicians. Given the small sample size at the single clinical setting, however, generalizability of these findings is limited.

Reading as a Woman/Doctoring as a Woman

This study adopted a feminist narrative model to differentiate women physicians' behavior from men physicians' behavior. The study postulated that the differences observed between women readers and men readers would be replicated in the interactional behaviors of women physicians and men physicians. Indeed, the gender differences among readers were replicated among doctors: women in both enterprises were more attentive to emotional and relational questions; they demonstrated greater skill in entering the narrative world of the "other" by appreciating the text on the one hand and recognizing life concerns of patients on the other. The women doctors acted as if they were alert to the emotional and daily life concerns of their patients, those concerns that tend to be muted in medical interactions, in a manner parallel to the woman reader's alertness to the implicit or muted aspects of women's texts. The women doctors exhibited interactional correlates to the attentiveness of the woman reader described by Hélène Cixous: despite exercising as much conversational control as men doctors, the women doctors were significantly more patient, engaged, egalitarian, and respectful of patients than were men. If nothing else, these findings suggest that medical training does not erase the specifically female ways of behaving from women doctors, as is sometimes feared.

Does this relatively complex analogic structure help to describe the characteristic attributes of the woman doctor and to postulate the sources of the differences between women and men doctors, or is the analogy to the woman reader merely a detour? It is hoped that adopting a feminist narrative model for the study of doctor-patient interactions emphasizes certain features of the interactions and offers a framework within which to make sense of the observations. Rather than achieving a set of fragmented findings about gender differences in medical practice, the model unifies the findings in a coherent pattern, suggesting further questions and research directions.

The findings reported here provisionally confirm the "fit" of the narrative model to the study of gender differences in doctor-patient interactions. Further implications of the model need to be articulated and studied, for the explanatory model's provisional usefulness will be confirmed only when its application prompts the raising and testing of fruitful questions.

Given the outlines of a phenomenon that can tentatively be called "doctoring as a woman," and applying Showalter's dictum about reading to doctoring, namely, that this enterprise is not confined to women, one can look specifically and directly for differences between men and women predicted by the model. Will the woman physician (or the man physician who has developed his skills in "doctoring as a woman") be better able than other physicians to ask Simone Weil's question, "What are you going through?" Will she be able to listen to the answer in a way that benefits her patients? Will mutuality in longitudinal medical relationships result in more clarity when patients face end-of-life decisions for themselves and their family members? Will attentiveness to gaps and silences in patient discourses or tolerance for silence result in the emergence of sets of concerns that remain hidden from physicians who practice otherwise? Might such attributes of women readers as discernment, ability to achieve critical detachment rather than dismissal, and ability to recognize seemingly disparate elements of a story be correlated to doctors' diagnostic or therapeutic capacities?

Adrienne Rich describes the power of reexamining texts in feminist studies: "Re-vision—the act of looking back, of seeing with fresh eyes, of entering an old text from a new critical direction—is for women more than a chapter in cultural history: it is an act of survival. Until we can understand the assumptions in which we are drenched we cannot know ourselves."[27] Doctors and those who study medicine are similarly engaged in a compelling search to make meaning out of a system of care that is losing its ability to address patients' true needs and offer true help. Examining medical relationships with feminist narrative frameworks may bare hidden assumptions and may help us to understand what, in fact, doctors ought to be able to do for patients. This is the effort under way, this is the cause, this is the longing.

Notes

1. Epigraph: Simone Weil, *Waiting for God*, trans. Emma Craufurd (London: Routledge & Kegan Paul, 1942), 59. The epigraph forms the dedication

for Adrienne Rich's poem "Leaflets" in Adrienne Rich, *The Facts of a Doorframe* (New York: W. W. Norton and Co., 1984), 99–104, 330.

2. See Debra Roter and Judith Hall, *Doctors Talking with Patients, Patients Talking with Doctors: Improving Communication in Medical Visits* (Westport, Conn.: Auburn House, 1992), for a review of recent research examining variables, including gender, that influence the patient-doctor relationship. Also see Debra Roter, Mack Lipkin, and A. Korsgaard, "Sex Differences in Patients' and Physicians' Communication during Primary Care Medical Visits," *Medical Care* 29 (1991):1083-1093. Candace West offers a conceptual model for examining women doctors' practice in "Reconceptualizing Gender in Physician-Patient Relationships," *Social Science and Medicine* 36 (1993):57–66. Also see Candace West, *Routine Complications: Troubles with Talk between Doctors and Patients* (Bloomington: Indiana University Press, 1984); Alexandra Dundas Todd, *Intimate Adversaries: Cultural Conflict between Doctors and Women Patients* (Philadelphia: University of Pennsylvania Press, 1989); Sherrie Kaplan, Sheldon Greenfield, and John Ware, "Assessing the Effects of Physician-Patient Interactions on the Outcomes of Chronic Disease," *Medical Care* 27 (1989):S110–127; Marie Haug and Marcia Ory, "Issues in Elderly Patient-Provider Interactions," *Research on Aging* 9 (1987):3–44; Ronald Adelman, Michele Greene, and Rita Charon, "Issues in Elderly Patient-Physician Interaction," *Ageing and Society* 11 (1991):127–148; and Mack Lipkin, Sam Putnam, and Aaron Lazare, eds., *The Medical Interview* (New York:Springer Verlag, in press).

3. Several investigators have criticized quantitative methodologies for lack of conceptual rigor. See David Tuckett and Anthony Williams, "Approaches to the Measurement of Explanation and Information-Giving in Medical Consultations: A Review of Empirical Studies," *Social Science and Medicine* 18 (1984):571–580; Thomas Inui and William Carter, "Problems and Prospects for Health Services Research on Provider-Patient Communication," *Medical Care* 23 (1985):521–538; Howard Waitzkin, "On Studying the Discourse of Medical Encounters: A Critique of Quantitative and Qualitative Methods and a Proposal for Reasonable Compromise," *Medical Care* 28 (1990):473–488; Candace West and Richard Frankel, "Miscommunication in Medicine," in *"Miscommunication" and Problematic Talk*, ed. Nikolas Coupland, Howard Giles, and John Weimann (Newbury Park, Calif.: Sage Publications, 1991), 166–194; and William Stiles, "Evaluating Medical Interview Process Components: Null Correlations with Outcomes May Be Misleading," *Medical Care* 27 (1989):212–220.

4. See Michele Greene, Ronald Adelman, Rita Charon, and Susie Hoffman, "Ageism in the Medical Encounter: An Exploratory Study of the Doctor–Elderly Patient Relationship," *Language and Communication* 6 (1986):113–124, for a description of the Geriatric Interaction Analysis instrument, which has, since its introduction, been modified to assess both doctors' and patients' interviewing behaviors and to be applicable to geriatric and nongeriatric medical encounters. The modified instrument has been renamed the Multi-Dimensional Interaction Analysis instrument.

5. Jerome Bruner, "The Narrative Constructions of Reality," *Critical Inquiry* 18 (1991):1–21, 4. See also Jerome Bruner, *Actual Minds, Possible Worlds* (Cambridge, Mass.: Harvard University Press, 1986); Bruner, *Reading for the Plot: Design and Intention in Narrative* (New York: Vintage Books, 1985); Wallace Martin, *Recent Theories of Narrative* (Ithaca: Cornell University Press, 1986); and Donald Polkinghorne, *Narrative Knowing and the Human Sciences* (Albany: State University of New York Press, 1988).

6. Medical work as a narrative enterprise has been described by Arthur Kleinman, *The Illness Narratives: Suffering, Healing, and the Human Condition* (New York: Basic Books, 1989); Howard Brody, *Stories of Sickness* (New Haven: Yale University Press, 1987; Robert Coles, *The Call of Stories: Teaching and the Moral Imagination* (Boston: Houghton Mifflin Company, 1989); and Eric J. Cassell, *Talking with Patients* (Cambridge, Mass.: MIT Press, 1985).

7. See Kathryn Hunter, *Doctors' Stories: The Narrative Structure of Medical Knowledge* (Princeton: Princeton University Press, 1991); and Rita Charon, "Medical Interpretation: Implications of Literary Theory of Narrative for Clinical Work," *Journal of Narrative and Life History* 3 (1993):79–97.

8. Barbara Herrnstein Smith, "Narrative Versions, Narrative Theories" in *On Narrative*, ed. W.J.T. Mitchell (Chicago: University of Chicago Press, 1981), 209–232, 228.

9. For the specific formulation of doctors' work as reading or as a hermeneutic enterprise, see Drew Leder, "Clinical Interpretation: The Hermeneutics of Medicine," *Theoretical Medicine* 11 (1990):9–24; Steven Daniel, "The Patient as Text: A Model of Clinical Hermeneutics," *Theoretical Medicine* 7 (1986):195–210; and Rita Charon, "Doctor-Patient, Reader-Writer: Learning to Find the Text," *Soundings* 72 (1989):137–152.

10. Wolfgang Iser, *The Act of Reading: A Theory of Aesthetic Response* (Baltimore: Johns Hopkins University Press, 1978), 19; Wolfgang Iser, *The Implied Reader: Patterns of Communication in Prose Fiction from Bunyan to Beckett* (Baltimore: Johns Hopkins University Press, 1974), 286, 275.

11. Reader-response criticism spans a wide continuum of theorists who describe the balance of power between texts and their readers. Early reader-response critics conceptualized the act of reading as a passive one in which the reader was taken up by the text and used for its purposes. See Georges Poulet, "Phenomenology of Reading," *New Literary History* 1 (1969):53–67. Critics such as Norman Holland and Stanley Fish suggest that the reader is the dominant source of meaning of a text, inflecting whatever is read with his or her characterological defenses and identity themes. See Norman Holland, *5 Readers Reading* (New Haven: Yale University Press, 1975); and Stanley Fish, *Is There a Text in This Class?* (Cambridge, Mass.: Harvard University Press, 1980). Such critics as Wolfgang Iser and Jonathan Culler locate the source of meaning in a dualistic interplay between text and reader. See Iser, *The Act of Reading: A Theory of Aesthetic Response*. A succinct summary of reader-response theories appears in Jonathan Culler, *On*

Deconstruction: Theory and Criticism after Stucturalism (Ithaca: Cornell University Press, 1982), 31–83.

12. See Judith Fetterley, *The Resisting Reader: A Feminist Approach to American Fiction* (Bloomington: Indiana University Press, 1978), for a discussion of the process of "immasculation," in which the woman reader, in face of the overwhelmingly male canon, not only is denied having her own experience legitimated but learns the lesson that "to be male—to be universal— . . . is to be *not female*" (xxiii).

13. Annette Kolodny, "A Map for Rereading: Gender and the Interpretation of Literary Texts," in *The New Feminist Criticism: Essays on Women, Literature, and Theory,* ed. Elaine Showalter (New York: Pantheon Books, 1985), 46–62.

14. Elaine Showalter, "Toward a Feminist Poetics," in *The New Feminist Criticism,* ed. Showalter, 125–143, 140, 142.

15. Sandra Gilbert and Susan Gubar, *The Madwoman in the Attic: The Woman Writer and the Nineteenth-Century Literary Imagination* (New Haven: Yale University Press, 1979), 75.

16. Quoted by Ann Rosalind Jones, "Inscribing Femininity: French Theories of the Feminine," in *Making a Difference: Feminist Literary Criticism,* ed. Gayle Greene and Coppelia Kahn (London: Routledge, 1986), 80–112, 94.

17. See Carol Gilligan, *In a Different Voice: Psychological Theory and Women's Development* (Cambridge, Mass.: Harvard University Press, 1982); and Carol Gilligan, Nona Lyons, Trudy Hanmer, eds., *Making Connections: The Relational Worlds of Adolescent Girls at Emma Willard School* (Cambridge, Mass.: Harvard University Press, 1990). See also Mary Field Belenky, Blythe McVicker Clinchy, Nancy Rule Goldberger, and Jill Mattuck Tarule, *Women's Ways of Knowing: The Development of Self, Voice, and Mind* (New York: Basic Books, 1986); Nel Noddings, *Caring: A Feminine Approach to Ethics and Moral Education* (Berkeley: University of California Press, 1984); and Sara Ruddick, *Maternal Thinking: Toward a Politics of Peace* (New York: Ballantine Books, 1989).

18. Adrienne Rich, *On Lies, Secrets, and Silence* (New York: W. W. Norton and Co., 1979), 159.

19. Patrocinio Schweickart, "Reading Ourselves: Toward a Feminist Theory of Reading," in *Gender and Reading: Essays on Readers, Texts, and Contexts,* ed. Elizabeth Flynn and Patrocinio Schweickart (Baltimore: Johns Hopkins University Press, 1986), 31–62, 47.

20. Although this is not the place to summarize the vast field of sources of gender differentiation, several of the major contributions can be enumerated. For discussions of the mother–daughter relationship, see Adrienne Rich, *Of Woman Born: Motherhood as Experience and Institution* (New York: W. W. Norton and Co., 1976); Dorothy Dinnerstein, *The Mermaid and the Minotaur: Sexual Arrangements and the Human Malaise* (New York: Harper & Row, 1976); Nancy Chodorow, *The Reproduction of Mothering: Psychoanalysis and the Sociology of Gender* (Berkeley: University of California Press, 1978); and Marianne Hirsch, "Mothers and Daughters," *Signs: Journal of Women in*

Culture and Society 7 (1981):200–222. For an analysis of gender differences in autobiographies, see Carolyn Heilbrun, *Writing a Woman's Life* (New York: Ballantine Books, 1988). Also see Nelly Furman, "The Politics of Language: Beyond the Gender Principle?" in *Making a Difference: Feminist Literary Criticism*, ed. Gayle Greene and Coppelia Kahn (London: Routledge, 1985), 59–79, for review. See also Mary Jacobus, *Reading Woman: Essays in Feminist Criticism* (New York: Columbia University Press, 1986), for an examination of feminist reading's ability to subvert patriarchal hierarchy.

21. Elizabeth Flynn, "Gender and Reading," *College English* 45 (March 1983): 236–253, 241, 247.

22. David Bleich, "Gender Interests in Reading and Language," in *Gender and Reading*, ed. Flynn and Schweickart, 234–266, 239.

23. Ibid., 239.

24. Chodorow, *The Reproduction of Mothering*, 110.

25. Flynn, "Gender and Reading," 237.

26. See Jonathan Culler, "Reading as a Woman," in Culler, *On Deconstruction*, 43–64, for a useful discussion of the interrelationship between reader-response theories and feminist approaches to texts.

27. Adrienne Rich, "When We Dead Awaken: Writing as Re-Vision," in Rich, *On Lies, Secrets, and Silence*, 35.

MARIAN GRAY SECUNDY

To Have a Heritage Unique in the Ages
Voices of African American Female Healers

The colored woman of today occupies . . . a unique position in this country. In a period of itself transitional and unsettled, her status seems one of the least ascertainable and definitive of all the forces which make for our civilization. She is confronted by both a woman question and a race problem. . . . But no woman can possibly put herself or her sex outside any of the interests that affect humanity. . . . She must stamp weal or woe on the coming history of this people. May she see her opportunity and vindicate her high prerogative.
Anna J. Cooper, *A Voice from the South*

Black feminism presumes the "intersectionality" of race and gender in the lives of black women, thereby rendering inapplicable . . . any "single-axis" theory about racism or sexism.
Valerie Smith, "Split Affinities: The Case of Interracial Rape"

Anna J. Cooper, educator and author, described her mission in life this way: "To have a heritage unique in the age," to "honor my name and vindicate my race."[1] The words of Cooper vividly come to mind when one examines the professional commitments of today's young women of color, particularly those who are physicians. These women occupy what is often called a borderland; they are "border cases" standing between the discourses of race and gender.[2] I was interested in how they have mediated these two cultural fields and how their situation frames their approach to doctor–patient communication.

Recently I interviewed nine African American female physicians to discover their views of themselves as care givers.[3] In an attempt to gain insight into the relationship between race, gender, class, and the capacity for empathy, these women were asked to describe their patients, their colleagues, their values—essentially, about what mattered to them in being physicians. I was curious to see what they might tell me about the experience of being black women professionals and to hear whether they viewed themselves as similar or dissimilar to their white female counterparts. I wondered, too, what they could tell me about their sense of self as women healers in contrast to the men with whom they work daily. The centrality of empathic responses and empathic care in the African American tradition is evident in their personal accounts. The interviews suggest, however, that these expressions of empathic awareness were elicited as much by shared experiences of culture and race as by the commonalities of gender.

Empathy is defined in English-language dictionaries as having both affective and cognitive aspects. Alfred Adler quoted an anonymous source as saying, "To empathize is to see with the eyes of another, to hear with the ears of another, and to feel with the heart of another."[4] From a clinical perspective, Douglas Olsen observes that an empathic clinician becomes immersed in the viewpoint of the patient.[5] J. Gagan speaks of "the ability to perceive the meanings and feelings of another person and to communicate that understanding to the other."[6] The *Encyclopedia of Psychology* states: "Empathy is generally understood to refer to one person's vicariously experiencing the feelings, perceptions, and thoughts of another."[7] Various theories suggest that the capacity for empathy is influenced by one's own psychological well-being, ego development, ego strength, and self-differentiation. Empathy requires the ability to accept the common humanity of the other. Carol Gilligan asserts that women's moral development emphasizes an ethic of care and relationship conducive to empathic response.[8] Olsen distinguishes between types of empathy. An empathic person can empathize with the cognitive world of "the other," with the affective world of "the other," with both, with a particular experience, and/or with a particular emotion. There is general agreement that one must have a positive view of "the other" to maximize one's empathic response or, at the very least, an ability to understand or make sense out of the experiences of "the other." These theories thus question the possibility of empathic responses in the absence of any of these capacities. They also raise the possibility that empathy based upon identification with "the other" might in some way become more inhibiting than enabling.

I accept definitions of empathy incorporating both the cognitive and the affective. I also believe that people are capable of responding empathically in a variety of ways. There are people who seem to be inherently empathic. Some, however, respond empathically only in technical, learned, and rehearsed ways. I claim that empathy is essentially a process and not merely a technique. Empathic behavior places one at risk of becoming too involved, losing objectivity, and becoming vulnerable to hurt. Sometimes an empathic response, at its core, requires behavior that appears on the surface to be harsh, *non*empathic. When one is empathic, however, the object of that empathy knows and understands that he/she is viewed as valuable and is cared about. Yet empathic responses can be learned, even when one is not feeling true empathy; sometimes, during moments of learned appropriate responses, one can be transformed. There is great power in the realization that care, when genuine, is perceived as such and that careful, attentive responses are better than noncareful, nonattentive ones. My conversations with interviewees demonstrated the varieties of empathy and empathic response.

Black women have been "buked" and have been scorned, in the words of the old Negro spiritual. They have been beasts of burden. They have been the nurturing mammies, nurses, maids, for millions of white children. They have been the kin keepers, the glue, the cement for their own people—for their men, for their children, and for each other. They have always, in the black vernacular, "been doin' it," and now, as we venture into the twenty-first century and look at our brown and black daughters, we strut with pride and grin foolishly at their magnificent accomplishments, at their articulations, their commitment to their people, at their determination to keep the faith and in so doing keep alive the dreams and legacies of all their mothers and grandmothers gone before. African American women physicians are no exception. Dr. Pamela Hollins, for example, recalls a white woman who called to complain that the community clinic was not properly controlling her maid Esther's blood sugar level. Dr. Hollins replied crisply to her caller that she, the white madam, could contribute more to Esther's health if she would pay her a living wage and provide health benefits so that Esther could afford her prescription drugs. Hollins laughs as she deplores the conditions under which "her" people have to live and die, because, at least on that one day, she, Dr. Pamela Hollins, age forty-one, internist, had struck a blow for humanity. But she also sighs in the telling, noting she could go on and on with tragic stories about applying Band-Aids when radical surgery, literally or figuratively, was necessary. Dr. Constance Holt, age fifty-eight, a family practitioner now employed by the Eastman Kodak Company in Rochester, New York, speaks of her need to engage in a people-oriented service profession and recalls the pain of losing a special patient after valiant efforts failed. She swallows hard, commenting, "It still haunts me, even today." Kathryn Moseley, neonatologist, thirty-six years old, Harvard educated, studying theology and ethics, writes from her Michigan base about a young mother of a fatally ill baby who told her, "You medical people are not perfect, because you don't take miracles into account." She says that it was through this experience that she learned that "things are not really as black and white as we practitioners portray; medicine is an art, not merely a science." The Chicago physicians Cheryl Woodson and Cynthia Henderson are geriatricians in their mid-thirties. Henderson talks of the importance of giving back some of the care she received as an ill child. Woodson, who trained at Wesleyan and the University of Pittsburgh, writes about the "special relationships" one develops with patients in longitudinal care. Omega Logan Silva's work as an administrative physician at the Veterans' Affairs Medical Center in Washington, D.C., causes her to reflect upon the legal, moral, and medical issues inherent in the use of life-sustaining technologies. Adrienne Mims, family physician, geriatrician, and administrator, attended Stanford Medical School and also holds a degree in public health from the University of California, Los Angeles. She cites as her reason for becoming a physician, "to improve the quality of medical care to lower-middle-class and poor African Americans." In her mid-thirties, Dr. Mims resides in Atlanta and struggles to recall any one memorable encounter with a patient, noting that *all* of her encounters have a special quality. Dr. Caryl Mussenden has quickly become, at forty, one of the most sought after obstetrician/gynecologists in the District of Columbia. She, like Drs. Holt and Silva, trained at Howard University College of Medicine and takes seriously Howard's charge to serve. She struggles with the new reproductive technologies and observes that, "my strong Christian faith has me questioning where to 'draw the line.'" September Williams, at thirty-six, has trained in internal medicine and specifically in hyperalimentation and critical care. Also a bioethicist and emergency care doctor in one of Chicago's busiest and bloodiest emergency rooms, she speaks simply of a calling "to be of service."

When asked their reasons for becoming physicians these women speak in much the same way as did their black female ancestors and in many of the same ways that Regina Morantz-Sanchez attributes to white women who entered the profession of medicine in the nineteenth century.[9] The themes are familiar: *a desire to be of service*, enjoyment of the intellectual challenge, an opportunity to improve the quality of medical care to the lower middle class and the poor, a wish for employment security, love of science, and a *desire to help others*. They do not speak with one voice, yet each response conveys something about the empathic orientation of these particular women. When asked her reason for entering the medical profession, Dr. Henderson responded simply that she was committed to care of the whole patient. Dr. Woodson spoke of the satisfaction in the special personal relationships one develops with patients and of her great desire to contribute to the training of physicians who care. Adrienne Mims wants to improve the quality of medical care of the lower middle class and of poor African Americans. She wants to be remembered as a physician who genuinely cared for, and listened to, her patients. Pamela Hollins entered the profession with the hope of improving some of the methods of health care delivery. She would like to be thought of as someone who "with God's grace, tried to provide high-quality health care for those who needed it the most but could least afford it." September Williams became a physician "to be of service" and to have the opportunity to have the people she touched professionally feel "elevated and respected" because of contact with her. Constance Holt spoke of wanting initially to be a nurse, always conscious of a need to engage in a service profession in which she could demonstrate genuine care and "make a difference."

Historically, as Darlene Clark Hine reminds us, the profession of nursing provided the one comparatively open gateway through which young black women of working-poor backgrounds could cross toward dignified employment and a middle-class lifestyle, while rendering much needed service to their people. As in the white community, access to careers for black women in nursing has been greater than access to careers in medicine. Hine notes that in some black communities nurses have been regarded as more responsive and sympathetic than doctors.[10] Midwives, too, have often been utilized in the absence of, and in preference to, physicians. The first black women physicians were graduated in the United States in 1864 and 1867, just a few years after emancipation and less than twenty years after the graduation of the first white woman physician. Rebecca Lee received her degree from the New England Female Medical College in 1864, followed by Rebecca J. Cole from the Woman's Medical College of Pennsylvania in 1867. Some, like Dr. Eliza Grier, entered the medical profession in the 1890s after having been slaves. By the 1920s more than two hundred black women physicians are known to have graduated from such medical schools as Meharry, Howard, and the Woman's Medical College. As of 1990, there were approximately 21,000 African American physicians in practice, of whom about 7,000 were female.[11]

Black female healers are unique in that they share the experiences of both racial oppression and gender discrimination. Currently and historically, their selection of public advocacy and public service as a primary career path has been one response to that common experience. Seven of the nine physicians interviewed hold or have held public service positions. Pamela Hollins has served as staff physician for a public health clinic in Baton Rouge, Louisiana; Cynthia Henderson is director of the geriatric medicine section of a long-term care facility in the city of Chicago; September Williams has worked in public health facilities throughout her career. There are clear patterns in the work of the earliest black women in medicine that can be identified today as well, including determination to escape poverty, desire for occupational mobility, self-fulfillment, fulfillment of parental and kin aspirations, altruism, service to humanity, a wish to help others, a desire to make a difference.

Like their professional ancestors, the women physicians I interviewed expressed concern both about critical problems facing the medical profession and the ethical problems they confront as individual physicians. The majority spoke eloquently about lack of access to care, rationing, cost containment, and differential care according to the patient's ability to pay. Their responses focused on their patients; insofar as they spoke of themselves or their profession, they did so in terms of the demoralization of physicians as a class owing to the effects of cost containment. They are advocates for change and, as Dr. Williams said, are becoming involved "in restructuring the health care system," building a new order that is "patient friendly."

These physicians expressed ethical concern over such issues as limited health care resources, health care rationing, and inadequate preparation for effectively treating patients of varying cultures. Prominent among their concerns were issues related to life-sustaining treatment, specifically advance directives and feeding tubes. Several women acknowledged personal concerns and conflicts regarding teenage pregnancy and reproductive rights. Some respondents revealed ambivalence toward their patients' behavior. At times they have experienced difficulty in responding empathically. Dr. Constance Holt described her anger and frustration with noncompliant and substance-abusing patients, although she acknowledges that social causes, external to the patients, contribute to many of their problems. Dr. Holt spoke of annoyance with sexually promiscuous teenagers, and supported the idea of stronger sanctions. As these women struggle with such issues, it is their self-awareness that makes empathic understanding possible.

Often they spoke of a need to give something back. When black women physicians talk of their patients, one also hears about their love of God, their commitment to their heritage, their responsibility to improve the common lot, to serve, and to care. They speak of a spiritual calling—one in which, in the words of the midwife Onnie Lee Logan, "the lord deal to me in visions to be a person to 'help somebody.'" She, like so many others, "asked God to help me."[12] As with Onnie Logan, these physicians tell about their love of the work and its relationship to the work of God. The importance of faith in God is ever present. Their recollections were studded with memories of mistreatment and the need to adopt coping behaviors. These healers, however, never seem to give up. They are strong women who keep on coming. Like the men in Sterling Brown's poetry, they are *strong women getting stronger*.[13]

The midwife Onnie Lee Logan remembered, "What I did was nothing but faith healing. And it wasn't all my faith. The patient had faith and I had faith and our faith went together."[14] Here, in this statement, we have the essence of empathy—mutuality and interactive understanding. Here there is no social construction of "the other" that places the healer above or beyond the arm's reach of those to whom she is ministering.

Although empathetic and caring, African American physicians often expressed that care as "tough love": they value self-improvement and race pride as much as responsiveness and understanding. Many black female healers have been misunderstood when they have been too assertive and directive, for although they care, they are, after all, health educators. When asked to discuss their most memorable encounters with patients, these physician respondents were unable to shed their clinical garb completely and talk nontechnically. They spoke of personal clinical triumphs and breakthroughs but in a somewhat more detached way than one might expect from other comments made about caring. It would appear that care and emotional expressiveness are not mutually dependent.

Nevertheless, although the impact of their clinical training is always apparent, personal concern for the patient and patient's family members was often expressed in ways that more scientific observers might find overly "subjective." The physicians interviewed spoke with feeling about the personal traumas associated with seriously ill or terminal patients. They remembered telling family members that they and the medical system had failed. Several of these modern-day doctors also spoke of their religious values as helpful in their capacity to deal with patients. They spoke of "miracles" and the unpredictability of prognosis. Caryl Mussenden tells of one especially difficult delivery. She takes pride in the fact that she did not panic and recalls it as a "truly satisfying experience." These experiences carry on the traditions of those many midwives of the early twentieth century who assisted in childbirth when no doctors were available, especially to the rural poor and black women of the South. As the "Granny midwife" Onnie Lee Logan recalled, "those old midwives . . . was black women not doin' it for a job but doin' it as a person knowin' there was need for it. They were doin' the very best they could to help . . . trying to help where the doctors didn't come around to help." The author Linda Janet Holmes tells us of hundreds of black lay midwives practicing in the deep South, some of whom had midwifery lineages that extended as far back as slavery. There were traditional black lay midwives, modern lay midwives, and nurse midwives. The traditional midwives acquired their skills empirically, following the paths of their grandmothers, mothers, or other senior midwives. Many of them were also known for their deep sense of spirituality. There is one particularly telling report by the midwife Mattie Hereford. Like Dr. Mussenden, she described an especially difficult delivery. Her celebratory prayer upon succeeding in birthing that particular baby was simply to say, "'Thank you, Jesus,' to myself."[15]

Dr. Omega Silva recalled important lessons learned from family members when the wife of an incurably ill man asked her to "let him die in peace." She noted that this "whole episode brought medical, ethical, and scientific issues into focus for me." What is evident is that this physician was able to hear and respond to her patient's wife in an empathic way. She came away from that experience convinced of the folly of undertaking procedures that can in no way better a patient's life.

Dr. Cheryl Woodson learned early as a second-year student the value of having a relationship with one's patients. She recalls that a patient asked for her opinion in the presence of "a famous vascular surgeon" and made it evident that she, the patient, trusted Dr. Woodson's word over "the great one" because "I had seen and talked to her daily, cared about what mattered to her (her diet, her bowels, her headaches, her grandchildren)."

In her memoir of becoming a physician, Dr. Vanessa Northington Gamble recalled one particularly difficult period in her training in the 1970s. She remembered, "One of the most painful reminders of my insecure status occurred during my junior clerkship in internal medicine. Wearing a lab coat and carrying a stethoscope, I walked into a patient's room at the Veterans' Affairs Hospital. The patient, an elderly white man, had been admitted for evaluation of a high blood calcium. I walked into his room and introduced myself as a student doctor. I proceeded to ask him questions about his medical history. Later, the white male intern came out of the patient's room. 'You know what that guy asked me?' he laughingly announced. 'Why didn't that girl clean up while she was in here?' My being mistaken for a maid became a joke on the ward team, all of whom, other than myself, were white and male."[16]

All nine female physicians I interviewed were asked to comment upon how they saw themselves as different from male practitioners, irrespective of race. All but one clearly expressed specific qualitative perceptions of difference.

Kathryn Moseley commented:

Having been a patient many times, and as a single mother with a child who has been ill, I believe I understand more and have a greater sense of compassion than male pediatricians. I think women have greater insight into parenting issues, and tend to be able to empathize more with patients: we talk to them and listen better, because we really care about the answers.

Caryl Mussenden described herself as much more compassionate than her male colleagues:

Being in my field [obstetrics/gynecology], I'm able to personally understand issues that my patients present to me. They seem comfortable in talking with me and frequently say they don't feel intimidated in discussing anything with me.

Constance Holt remarked:

Firstly, I trust my appearance clearly identifies me as a feminine woman, in the traditional sense. Secondly, it's been my experience that women do, indeed, bring some special qualities (needed ones) to the art of medicine. Women usually are more inclined to be patient (not always the case with male physicians) in situations which call for patience rather than action. Women generally are more likely to consider the female point of view on questions rather than automatically going to the traditional (male) response.

Pamela Hollins noted:

Comparatively speaking, I rely on intuitive feelings in assessing clinical problems more than my male counterparts. I have had a great deal of success doing this. I tend to probe deeper into the patient's true reasons for seeking medical attention. I also utilize community support agencies more in a case plan. Many clinical problems cannot be adequately addressed until nonclinical problems are identified and managed.

Adrienne Mims stated that she sees herself as more nurturing and more sincere than her male colleagues:

I think I am more sensitive, prone to listen with a third ear, for unsaid issues and background; look with a third eye at how the whole picture fits; tend more to pay attention to little, minor details that make the difference.

Omega Silva sees herself as a better all-around physician than most males. September Williams perceives differences because she sees her responsibility to her family, to the arts, and to all humanity as *equal* to her sense of professional responsibility, implying that the majority of males do not.

The nine female physicians were asked, finally, to comment upon how they saw themselves as different from white physicians, male and female. Every woman noted very specific differences when asked about their white colleagues—female as well as male. In fact none of them, interestingly enough, made any distinction between white men and white women. Here it is important to keep in mind the collective consciousness of racism of which we spoke earlier. White women have also been oppressors of black people, including black women, even as they, themselves, were oppressed. They, too, have erected personal and professional barriers.[17]

Adrienne Mims described herself as more considerate and empathic than her white colleagues—male and female. Kathryn Moseley stated:

I'm more "wonderful" because I'm less rigid and closed. White physicians, in my experience, tend to be rather compulsive about maintaining a definite bridge between patient and physician. I think patients, black and white, have a greater sense of comfort with black practitioners. They feel greater freedom to engage in conversations not related to their problems. As a patient, I have found this more easy-going practice style far more common among black physicians than white. It seems to have something to do with respect. You don't find black doctors calling a sixty-year-old black woman patient by her first name while insisting on being addressed as Dr. So-and-So. White physicians do that all the time.

Constance Holt responded:

Because Afro-Americans have historically been given second-rate care by many health care providers of the majority group, this has added to the anxiety of many who have to deal regularly with health care systems which are not sensitive to their cultural needs. As a practitioner, my experience has been made rich many times over when I have seen and felt that being there for my people has made all the difference to and for them.

Dr. Cynthia Henderson observed, "I make fewer assumptions about ethnic and cultural backgrounds and how they affect patient understanding and compliance."

Cheryl Woodson, however, commented that she thinks the differences are not gender or race related, but based on personal values and "home training." She states:

> I have seen physicians of both sexes and all ethnic backgrounds who had excellent "bedside manners" and the same mixture of people who had no respect for patients outside some laboratory. More scary were the physicians and trainees who simply lacked skill in interpersonal relations, neither actively disrespecting nor interacting positively. My greatest concern is that medical training fails to focus on interpersonal skills. Because of this, those of us who retain this value do so serendipitously and despite the training. Medical education must emphasize "people skills" as well as medical science.

Dr. Silva tended to agree with Dr. Woodson, although noting that her own experiences as a black person might shape the health care she provides to others. And September Williams said, "I feel with my patients; I am not separate from them."

There is no specific identification by these particular black women with women physicians as a distinct class or category. Their sense of concern for all patients, their perceptions of themselves as caring, nurturing, empathic people is apparent in what these women say about themselves. We can only assume that their patients would agree with them.

African American female physicians essentially defy traditional stereotypes. As our group attests, their backgrounds are varied; their motivations are multifaceted; their personalities are unique. It is not possible to make conclusive statements about the intersection of race and gender from these brief historical accounts and interviews. Much more detailed analysis, larger samples, and comparative research are necessary for such determinations.

But at this juncture, reported patient perceptions, self reports, and empirical observations do, of course, give us some significant information. Black female physicians do appear to express their caring and nurturing predilections in ways less apparent in other physicians. At least they certainly perceive themselves that way. Other variables that may also influence these healers' capacities for empathy—family and personality characteristics, age, impact of medical education, choice of medical specialty, for example—need more careful exploration. As women are viewed and treated in more egalitarian ways, they may find it unnecessary to cultivate and foster nurturance and caring as primary values. Echoing the theories of Carol Gilligan, however, we do in fact hear a nurturing, holistic model of interaction through these voices. These particular female healers are speaking "in a different voice." Their primary experiences are experiences of attachment and affiliation to others, as Gilligan suggests they usually are. One continues to wonder, with social scientists, if gender differences in moral and social sensibilities result merely from social status and socialization. If, as Morantz-Sanchez asks, a truly gender-neutral society were achieved, would these different moral and social sensibilities disappear?[18]

Black female healers do not appear to have consciously struggled with gender issues as much as they have with issues of race and oppression. In 1972 Cynthia Fuchs Epstein studied thirty-one black women professors, including lawyers, physicians, university professors, and executives. She discovered that achievement was strongly associated with the attitude of each woman's family, her sense of self worth, the role of her mother, and her superior's conception of her. The mothers of these women were doers; most of the mothers had worked outside the home. The evidence suggests that the female healers I interviewed had similar patterns.[19] Most of them have succeeded out of sheer dogged determination and persistence. Joyce Ladner reminds us in *Tomorrow's Tomorrow*, "Black womanhood has always been the very essence of what American womanhood is attempting to become on some levels."[20]

As Patricia Hill Collins comments, there are at least three components of the African American woman's ethic of caring: the value placed on individual expressiveness, a belief in the appropriateness of emotional expression, and the capacity for empathy that pervades African American culture. There would appear to be, as Collins suggests, some convergence of Afrocentric and feminist values in the ethics of care (and empathy), but as she also notes, "While white women may have access to a women's tradition valuing emotion and expressiveness, few white social institutions except the family validate this way of knowing."[21] Black institutions, in contrast, particularly the church, reflect the deep roots of the African past along with the black family.

Collins, in her discussion of the social construction of black feminist thought, makes several other critical observations. She describes the distinctive interpretations that black women have given to their oppression and to the oppression of their people. She also discusses the alternative ways used by black women to produce and validate knowledge, especially empathic processes and skills. Collins's observations seem to be illustrated by the oral narratives of the African American female healers I interviewed. Most of these women appear to have resisted relating to patients in the language of "scientific objectivity" where this would entail distance, detachment, or manipulation.

Emotional expression is not absent from their patient encounters or their descriptions of their work. Concrete experience informs their behavior and interpretations of meaning: "Distant statistics are certainly not as important as the actual experience of a sober person."[22] Thomas Kochman describes situations in which every verbal communication between blacks assumes active participation of at least two human beings, the speaker and the listener.[23] We find this, too, in the reported interactive processes of these African American healers with their patients and the communities to which they minister. Talking with your heart is valued. Personal expressiveness, emotions, and empathy are priorities. The ethic of personal accountability pervades African American culture and the stories of these women as well: one's personal life ought to be consistent with one's espoused values. According to a favorite black expression, responsibility is "putting your body where your mouth is."

Female African American healers would appear to have a clear understanding of, and significant capacity for, empathic responses to those for whom they care. In addition to sharing the commonality of gender, these black women healers have shared a common history of racism and oppression in this country that, they tell us, has shaped who they are. Some scholars also claim the significance of a collective consciousness of Africanist traditions and customs. I believe both to be operative. As Sandra Harding observes, gender and race are social and, therefore, historical categories.[24]

Much work is yet to be done in analysis, comparative research, and identification of critical variables. Exploring the connections between the moral development of white women and black women necessitates further explication and much more detailed comparative research. The tapestry is being woven. Hearing the voices of female African American healers is, indeed, just a beginning.

Notes

1. First epigraph: As quoted in Dorothy Sterling, *We Are Sisters* (New York: W. W. Norton and Co., 1984), 450; second epigraph: Valerie Smith, "Split Affinities: The Case of Interracial Rape," in *Conflicts in Feminism*, ed. Marianne Hirsch and Evelyn Fox Keller (New York: Routledge, 1990), 272; Cooper quotation: Sterling, *We Are Sisters*, 449.

2. Valerie Smith discusses as "border cases" those sites where "ideologies of racial and gender differences come into tension with and interrogate each other," 272.

3. Interviews were conducted with the following female physicians:

Internist	September Williams, M.D.	Chicago, Ill.
Internist	Constance Holt, M.D.	Rochester, N.Y.
Family Physician	Adrienne Mims, M.D.	Atlanta, Ga.
Pediatrician	Kathryn Moseley, M.D.	Detroit, Mich.
Geriatrician	Cynthia Henderson, M.D.	Chicago, Ill.
Ob/Gyn	Caryl Mussenden, M.D.	Washington, D.C.
Internist	Pamela Hollins, M.D.	Baton Rouge, La.
Internist	Omega Silva, M.D.	Washington, D.C.
Geriatrician	Cheryl Woodson, M.D.	Chicago, Ill.

4. Quoted in Douglas Olsen, "Empathy as an Ethical and Philosophical Basis for Nursing," in *Adv. Nurs. Sci.* 14:1 (1991):63. Citation from R. L. Katz, *Empathy: Its Nature and Uses* (London: Collier-Macmillan, 1963).

5. Douglas Olsen, "Empathy as an Ethical and Philosophical Basis," 65.

6. J. Gagen, "Methodologic Notes on Empathy," *ANS* 5:2 (1983):65–72.

7. R. Corsine, ed., The Encyclopedia of Psychology (New York: Wiley, 1984), 428.

8. Carol Gilligan, *In a Different Voice: Psychological Theory and Women's Development* (Cambridge, Mass.: Harvard University Press, 1982).

9. Regina Morantz-Sanchez, *Sympathy and Science: Women Physicians in American Medicine* (New York: Oxford University Press, 1985), 358.

10. Darlene Clark Hine, *Black Women in White* (Bloomington: Indiana University Press, 1989), xix, xxi.

11. Darlene Clark Hine, "Co-Laborers in the Work of the Lord: Nine-teenth-Century Black Women Physicians," in *"Send Us a Lady Physician": Women Doctors in America, 1835–1920*, ed. Ruth Abrams (New York: W. W. Norton and Co., 1985), 107; "Minorities in Medicine," *Science* 258 (1992):1087. For the following 1990 figures we are indebted to Jeanne Benetti of the U.S. Census Bureau, personal communication with Ellen More.

Editorial note: In 1992, 782 black female applicants were admitted to American medical schools, an increase of 20 percent over 1991. The number of males admitted in 1992 was 509, only a slight increase over 1991. As of 1990 the ratio of male to female black physicians was only 2:1 (13,707 versus 7,167) compared with a male-female ratio of more than 3:1 overall.

12. Onnie Lee Logan, *Motherwit* (New York: Plume, 1989), 67.

13. Sterling A. Brown, "The Collected Poems of Sterling A. Brown," in *Strong Men*, ed. Michael Harper (New York: Harper & Row, 1983), 56.

14. Logan, *Motherwit*, 145.

15. Ibid., p. 65. See also Linda Janet Holmes, "'Thank You Jesus to Myself.' The Life of a Traditional Black Midwife," in *The Black Women's Health Book: Speaking for Ourselves*, ed. Evelyn White (Seattle: The Seal Press, 1990), 98–107.

16. Vanessa Northington Gamble, "On Becoming a Physician: a Dream Not Deferred," in *The Black Women's Health Book*, ed. White, 52–65.

17. For historical accounts of these painful relations, see Hine, "Co–Laborers in the Work of the Lord," 112; Sterling, *We Are Sisters,* 160.

18. Morantz-Sanchez, *Sympathy and Science,* 60.

19. Cynthia Fuchs Epstein, "Positive Effects of the Double Negative: Explaining the Success of Black Professional Women," *American Journal of Sociology* (1972):919.

20. Joyce Ladner, *Tomorrow's Tomorrow* (Garden City, N.Y.: Doubleday, 1971), 127.

21. Patricia Hill Collins, "The Social Construction of Black Feminist Thought," in *Black Women in America,* by Micheline Malson et al. (Chicago: University of Chicago Press, 1988), 320.

22. Ibid.

23. Thomas Kochman, *Black and White Styles in Conflict* (Chicago: University of Chicago Press, 1981), 111.

24. Sandra Harding, "The Curious Coincidence of Feminine and African Moralities: Challenges for Feminist Theory," in *Women and Moral Theory,* ed. Eva Feder Kittay and Diana T. Meyers (Totowa, N.J.: Rowman & Littlefield Publishers, 1987), 296–315.

JANET BICKEL

Special Needs and Affinities of Women Medical Students

If women . . . articulate a perspective which links achievement with attachment, women physicians may help to heal the breach in medicine between patient care and scientific success. For this reason the encouragement of women's voices and the validation of women's perceptions may contribute to the improvement of medical education. Since humanism in medicine depends on joining the heroism of cure with the vulnerability of care, reshaping the image of the physician to include women constitutes a powerful force for change.

Carol Gilligan and Susan Pollack

The proportion of medical students who are women has grown from 6 percent in 1960 to 25 percent in 1980 to 39 percent in 1993.[1] Although there is some evidence that women bring certain affinities to medicine, for instance in communicating with patients, findings relative to gender differences are often difficult to interpret and substantiate. For one thing, women are just as diverse as men. Another problematic feature of special claims for women is that such claims can reinforce the expectation that women physicians will remain the "worker bees" of clinical care, while men continue to dominate the more prestigious and policy-shaping areas of medicine.

But studies reveal that certain gender-related differences do exist and may stand in the way of women's fullest participation in medicine. These ought to be addressed. Moreover, if these differences represent potential strengths that women bring to medicine, exploring these issues may work to strengthen medical education and practice.

The following will highlight recent findings pertaining to gender differences in medical education, with particular attention to barriers to the development of empathic communication skills. The work of Jean Baker Miller is relevant here. Miller has observed that our culture encourages men to develop the qualities of separateness, achievement, and aggression while encouraging women to develop the qualities of connection, caring, and accommodation.[2] If women more than men students tend to bring this higher valuing of and need for connection to medical school, they also have more to lose from the dehumanizing aspects of the educational experience. But, as the essays in this volume indicate, work to improve the gender climate in medical education will help both sexes to become more empathic physicians.

Differences between Men and Women Medical Students

The Association of American Medical Colleges (AAMC) maintains a national student database that allows comparison of men and women matriculants' responses to a large variety of demographic, education-related, and attitudinal variables. Overall, men and women students are much more alike than different. In results from 1991, however, women expressed slightly less confidence than did men in their ability to succeed in medical school (66 percent of women versus 75 percent of men say they are "very confident"). Of students planning a salaried or private practice, 59 percent of women and 74 percent of men predict they will be a specialist (as distinct from a family physician or general pediatrician). Men more than women also tend to place more importance on "high income possibilities" and "status and prestige" relative to medicine as a career goal. With regard to the physician service considered most important, 45 percent of women compared with 31 percent of men select "working with patients to *prevent* illness."

In response to the AAMC's Medical School Graduation Questionnaire (GQ), women seniors express more dissatisfaction than men with their education.[3] In 1992, more women than men ranked as "inadequate" the curriculum time devoted to twenty-five of the twenty-seven areas named, with the greatest gender differences in the evaluation of effective patient education, management of patients' socioeconomic and emotional problems, cost-effective medical practice, and use of computers. This consistent finding probably reflects a combination of lower levels of self-confidence; higher expectations regarding the quality of their education, particularly in the areas of preventive medicine and managing those patient needs that extend beyond the strictly biomedical arena; and the likelihood that a predominantly male faculty is more comfortable with men than women students. An extensive report issued by the American Association of University Women found that whether one looks at preschool classrooms or university lecture halls, at male or female teachers, research spanning the past twenty years consistently reveals that males receive more teacher attention than do females.[4]

Another GQ question related to the medical school experience that elicited substantial gender difference was "Have you ever been sub-

jected to sexual harassment or discrimination while in medical school?";
60 percent of women and 14 percent of men said "yes." With regard to
the form the discrimination took, men most commonly noted favorit-
ism, poor evaluations, perceived hostility, and denied opportunity. Although sizable proportions of women also reported these forms of
discrimination, three times more women than men reported sexist slurs,
sexist teaching materials, and sexual advances. These results have been
corroborated by studies of student mistreatment conducted at individual medical schools, for instance, by K. H. Sheehan and colleagues.[5]
Even more recently a study of the mental health consequences of medical student abuse found that students reporting at least one abusive
experience were more likely than others to experience depressive symptoms and to use alcohol to escape. This study found that 77 percent of
women and 69 percent of men experienced some form of abuse, which
was, however, rather broadly defined; for example, "I have experienced discomfort listening to sexual humor." Women were more likely
than men to report exclusions from informal settings, discomfort from
sexual humor, and unwanted sexual advances.[6]

In another enduring area of concern, AAMC Graduate Questionnaire
results substantiate that residency program directors ask women personal questions more frequently than men. Women were much more
likely than men to be asked about the stability of their interpersonal
relations and their intention to have children. Sometimes these family-
related inquiries became the focus of an interview; it is not surprising
that women were not asked as frequently as men about their career
plans. Women were five times more likely to be questioned about their
commitment to medicine, however, and twice as likely to be asked
about their spouse's support for their decision to pursue medical training. Women were also seven times more likely than men to report the
occurrence of an offensive incident during their interview.

In the area of academic ability, the performance of men and women
medical students is for the most part indistinguishable.[7] Men medical
students tend to perform better on standardized knowledge-based
achievement tests while women do better in person-related tasks.[8] On
the National Board of Medical Examiners, Part I (covering the sciences
basic to medicine), women tend to score lower than men, but on Part II
(clinical sciences) women tend to score higher. A 1992 study by R. J.
Paimes and colleagues found that only in the pediatrics clerkship did
women outperform men in all three areas: mini-Boards, faculty evaluation, and overall grade.[9]

Efforts to improve the evaluation of students' clinical skills are leading to the increased use of standardized patients (SP). Interestingly,

two studies looking at the influence of student and SP gender on performance-based clinical examinations found that men and women students performed equally.[10]

Given the complexities of moral orientation and moral reasoning, the
evaluation of qualities associated with moral development remains controversial, and few studies of medical students have been published.
Rest's Defining Issues Test (DIT), which presents six moral dilemmas
on which the scoring is justice-oriented, was administered to students
at one midwestern medical college.[11] Contrary to the contention of
Carol Gilligan that women generally score lower on this type of moral
reasoning test,[12] for every medical school class, the women's moral
reasoning scores were higher than men's. The authors do not find these
results surprising, given that many women medical students exhibit
other characteristics traditionally associated with male behavior (for
example, competitiveness), but additional studies of medical students
are needed before firm conclusions can be drawn.

Many studies have found differences in how men and women medical trainees experience and deal with stress, and most of these find that
women experience more psychological distress than do men.[13] One
recent study, however, found that, as measured on the Profile of Mood
States, women residents did not experience a higher level of emotional
distress than men, probably because they more frequently used social
support and positive reappraisals as coping strategies.[14] Another study
found that, while women seek psychiatric consultation twice as often
as do men students, women do not remain in treatment longer than
men. This study also found that women with dependent personality
disorder—that is, strong internalization of the traditional female role—
usually experience severe role-related conflicts during medical school.[15]

As part of a longitudinal study of stress in physicians, Gilligan and
Pollack examined the responses of first-year medical students to the
Thematic Apperception Test (TAT). Their results are of particular interest. In stories written in response to pictures, one-third of men but no
women associated *intimacy* with danger. While no men linked *isolation*
with danger, 44 percent of the women did. The authors conclude that
women's perceptions about the healing power of relationships and their
vigilance to the dangers of detachment help to explain the greater stress
they experience. Moreover, "Women medical students in their heightened sensitivity to detachment and isolation often reveal the places in
medical training and practice where human connection has become
dangerously thin. Women's concerns about connection, however, may
also invoke the specter of disconnection, with the result that women
may be reluctant to initiate conflict and change."[16]

F. W. Hafferty's study of first-year medical students' reactions to human dissection and to terminally ill patients contributes relevant findings here as well, even though gender differences were not part of the initial study focus. The women students were better able than the men to deal with situations involving ambiguity, more reflective about their own reactions to situations, more aware of the reactions of others, and better able to anticipate how emotionally taxing certain situations might be. Thus they emerged as more supportive and empathetic when peers expressed concerns. This study consistently found that women medical students of all ages appeared to be more sensitive to the emotions of others and more comfortable with a language of emotions than men. Hafferty hypothesizes that a primary reason for the women's comfort with emotion is that a posture of detached indifference is not expected of women to the same degree that it is of men. Nonetheless, he concludes that in medical education "the predominant trend [is] the reinforcement of the norms of detached indifference and emotional control." Pressures remain high for women in medicine to appear unemotional and tough. Both this study and the one by Gilligan and Pollack lead to the observation that women may indeed bring to the healing relationship a readier capacity for empathy than do men, but that medical training likely attenuates it. Moreover, Hafferty concludes that "it remains painfully obvious that the male domination of medicine continues to exert a toll not only on patients and practitioners, but on the profession as well."[17]

Yet, despite more gender discrimination and harassment, more role conflicts, fewer same-sex role models, and more dissatisfaction with the curriculum, women students overall perform as well as men. In fact, in some clinical areas, women outperform men. Another observation, given the results of the TAT and of other studies of medical students, is that women seem more aware of the losses resulting from the depersonalization often found in medical education. Nonetheless, the work of reducing medical education's dehumanizing aspects demands the best efforts of both sexes.

Career- and Specialty-Related Differences

With regard to specialty choice, although there has been a decline in the proportions of both sexes entering primary care areas, the distribution of men and women across specialties has not changed very much. In 1985, 68 percent of practicing women physicians and 44 percent of men worked in primary care fields.[18] On the 1992 AAMC Graduate Questionnaire, 62 percent of women and 45 percent of men responded affirmatively to the question, "Do you plan to devote all or part of your practice to primary care?" With regard to plans to become certified in specific specialties, an equal or greater proportion of women than men students choose the primary care areas: 19 percent of both sexes plan on internal medicine, 12 percent of women and 10 percent of men on family practice, 17 percent of women and 5 percent of men on pediatrics, and 14 percent of women and 6 percent of men on obstetrics/ gynecology. When women and men were asked about factors positively influencing their specialty choices, though their ranking of many factors was quite similar, women were more influenced than men by "strong emphasis on patient education and prevention," "emphasis on people skills rather than technical skills," and by "strong emphasis on primary care"; men gave a higher ranking than women to "income" and "prestige." When asked about plans to locate their practices in a socioeconomically deprived (SED) area, 14 percent of women seniors and 8 percent of men, checked "yes."

Corroborating these findings is a study linking AAMC and AMA data which found that 46 percent of women compared with 35 percent of men who as seniors predicted a primary care practice, actually did follow through. This study also showed that with regard to practice in a SED area, women were twice as likely as men to be treating poor people, and women were twice as likely as men to have followed through on their plans for this kind of practice.[19] Another recent study with practice implications found that women medical students were more willing than men to treat AIDS patients.[20]

If we keep in mind Gilligan and Pollack's TAT results that suggest that women more than men desire closer communication with patients, it is not surprising that a higher percentage of women enter primary rather than more procedure-based care. Related evidence here comes from a study of Quebec general practitioners: the women physicians were more likely than men to value psychosocial factors in patient care, patient education, and health counseling.[21] Structural factors also predispose women toward primary care. Child care responsibilities, for example, often play a greater role in women's than in men's career decisions; and the climate in this regard is more positive in pediatrics and family medicine than, for example, in surgery. Likewise, the shorter training period for generalists compared with specialists is important for some parents. Another influence is certainly the comparatively higher number of women mentors in primary care fields. For example, in 1993 the proportion of faculty who were women in pediatrics, family medicine, and surgery was 37, 29, and 10 percent, respectively.[22]

With regard to specialty choice, recent studies also sound some cautionary notes. Paimes and colleagues found that, although only 8 percent of women students indicated an interest in pediatrics upon matriculation, one third of them entered a pediatrics residency.[23] Because these investigators also found that women's specialty choices were more influenced by faculty evaluations than were men's, these results suggest that some faculty may be "pigeon-holing" some women. Another study comparing men and women's experiences on a surgery clerkship found that although men scored higher on the in-house and NBME examinations, women received better performance ratings from faculty, and no gender-related differences were found in their performance as first-year residents. Only half as many women as men, however, entered surgery residencies. Students were asked to rate fifteen aspects of the clerkship; women gave twelve of these lower ratings than did the men. The authors conclude that if women's surgery clerkship experience were equivalent to men's in terms of attitudes of staff and skill development opportunities, more women would be likely to enter surgery.[24]

A final relevant study to cite with regard to career choice is an investigation of young physicians most and least likely to have second thoughts about a medical career. J. Hadley and colleagues found that, two to six years out of residency, white women and blacks and Hispanics of both sexes reported the greatest reservations. These investigators conclude that a better understanding is needed of how women and minority students are being steered toward or away from particular specialties and how they are made to feel uncomfortable in participating in the full spectrum of medical training opportunities.[25]

That women more often than men enter primary care and care for the underserved is a boon to the American health care system. Nonetheless, efforts should focus on assuring that women have access to the same skill development opportunities and range of specialty choices that men take for granted. In any case, looking to women physicians to solve the country's health care imbalances would be misguided. The best efforts of both sexes are needed to improve patients' access to primary care and to empathic care. Another point is that women make excellent surgeons just as they make excellent pediatricians; a more varied distribution of women physicians is desirable because patient demand for women physicians exists in every specialty. Moreover, women's research efforts, in addition to their care-giving skills, are needed in every area.

Current Barriers in Medical Education

That many features of medical education are far from ideal for shaping empathic physicians is obvious. An analysis of these features is beyond the scope of this essay, but three issues deserve comment because of their particular impact on women.

First, since at least the late eighteenth century, medicine has glorified what can be measured and devalued affective aspects of experience. A great deal of both patient dissatisfaction and physician impairment can be traced to an educational system that overemphasizes the importance of detachment, abstraction, and the technical at the expense of the emotive and communicative aspects of patient care. That much of medical education occurs in large groups and lacks a personal touch contributes here as well; students can graduate without any one faculty member or dean getting to know them well. But as Janet Surrey and Stephen Bergman also ask in their essay, how can students learn to care for patients as individuals if no one is caring about them as individuals? If the findings of Gilligan and Pollack and Hafferty are correct, it seems likely that medical education's depersonalizing effects exact more of a toll from women than from men.[26]

Second, throughout society, women more than men have suffered the effects of sexism and gender bias. Because sexual harassment is more about power than sex and because of the authority that doctors enforce over students and all other members of the health care team, problems with sexism may be more pronounced in medicine than in many other sectors. The rigid educational hierarchy, evaluation pressures, long hours, and focus on the human body are also potent influences in this regard.

Conscious and unconscious slights and other such "microinequities" have widespread effects.[27] Carola Eisenberg writes, "The credentials of women are subtly discounted because of prejudice so thoroughly inculcated in men (and in all too many women) that it operates automatically, often altogether without awareness."[28] Examples abound. Women professionals report being referred to by their first names while the men in the room are addressed as "doctor." Women are subject to comments downplaying their professional commitment while focusing undue attention on their appearance. When being evaluated on a clerkship or for tenure, a woman may be called "overly aggressive" when in a man the same behavior would be labeled "forceful" or "strong." Hafferty illustrates how to be "tough enough" to survive many rites of passage without becoming hardened presents continuing challenges to both sexes, but especially to women.[29] Because women students have far fewer same-sex role models and because women in our society are allowed a far narrower band of assertive behavior than are men ("womanliness" still is associated with submissive qualities), discovering effective coping and negotiating strategies remains a lonely process.

Third, parenting responsibilities create a need for more flexible structures and timetables than academia customarily provides. With arrangements structured primarily for men with domestic supports, women in the professions and in most workplaces continue to be penalized for having children. And because few "pause" buttons are built into academic medicine's long continuum, improvements here (such as parental leave, flexible benefits) lag behind the private sector.

It is not known how many medical students have children during medical school, but 88 percent of women and 87 percent of men seniors responding to the GQ in 1992 reported zero children; those who enter medical school with children or acquire them during that interval remain a fairly small minority. Most women who enter medicine, however, eventually combine medicine with parenting. The most recent study of women medical school faculty showed that 79 percent of those who had ever been married had children.[30]

Medical students who are parents, especially single parents, often have greater needs for flexibility in course scheduling and for financial aid than other students. Thus student-parents at institutions with a lock-step curriculum and where affordable child care is scarce may find it difficult to manage. Most academic medical centers do not offer child care services, and when they do, access for medical students is limited by long waiting lists and high fees. Another parenting-related dilemma facing medical students is whether to lie during their residency interviews regarding childbearing hopes, since few program directors welcome pregnant residents. (In 1991, the AAMC published a resource for medical students, residents, faculty and program directors to help address these issues.)[31] Focused mainly on meeting service needs, program directors tend to discount the biomedical knowledge and other care-giving and administrative skills that physicians acquire as parents.

Desirable Institutional Responses

Any change that improves the environment for women will also benefit men, because it will be in the direction of humanizing the institution. A more humane educational environment will produce more empathic care givers and better learners. Certainly the best-led medical schools are continuously engaged in improving their educational programs in a variety of ways. The following are just a few examples of programs particularly responsive to the needs outlined above.

• Because as a medical student he had felt little support for dealing with the emotional impact of patient care or with personal crises, when Doyle Graham, M.D., served as dean of Duke University School of Medicine, he created the "advisory dean system." He had learned about the benefits of support largely from participating in men's groups, where he gained experience in relating to other men as friends rather than as potential competitors. The advisory dean system is based on four associate deans, each of whom is assigned a quarter of each class on admission and remains the group's dean until graduation. In regular groups of about ten, students meet weekly during the first year (less frequently thereafter), with discussions focusing on values and other issues of immediate concern to the students. In addition to being deliberately nurturant and to providing a supportive community, this system allows better evaluation of students and better personal and professional counseling.

• Women's health is gaining prominence nationally (for example, in 1990 the National Institutes of Health created the Office for Research on Women's Health) and at a number of medical schools. McMaster University Faculty of Health Sciences established a Women's Health Office in 1991. The definition of women's health promulgated by this office includes the emotional, social, cultural, spiritual, and economic context of women's lives. Women faculty who teach women's health electives at Brown University School of Medicine, University of Pennsylvania School of Medicine, and Dartmouth-Hitchcock Medical Center are also broadening the traditional conception of women's health to include greater application of the biopsychosocial model. Such efforts also help to counter trainees' perceptual biases about women as patients, with positive effects on the gender climate overall.

• With regard to parenting and flexibility issues, at least fifteen schools have lengthened their tenure probationary period beyond the traditional seven years, which is likely to ease unnecessary time pressures for some faculty. Yale University School of Medicine and University of Pennsylvania School of Medicine have made it possible to remain on tenure track with a part-time appointment. The Medical College of Wisconsin relabeled its part-time option "full-time professional effort" and enhanced this option in a number of ways—for example, malpractice coverage is paid by the department. Beth Israel Hospital in Boston remains the best example of a comprehensive approach to meeting the needs of parents, including on-site child care, a breastfeeding support program, and flexible scheduling and benefits.

• Stanford University Medical School's dean's office and Women in Medicine Committee have developed a multifaceted approach to eliminating sexism, including retreats for women faculty and students and required gender sensitivity training for department chairs and senior faculty.

In order to introduce long-term, far-reaching improvements in the gender climate, ideally the dean, other senior administrators, and an organized group of women faculty and students need to work together to develop strategies for change.[32] The AAMC's Women in Medicine program aims to help schools with this work and with increasing the number of women moving into positions of leadership in academic medicine. Academic medicine needs women in senior positions as role models for students and also for the perspective and commitment to progress they can bring to the policymaking table. Sidney Callahan notes, "Creativity comes from having been outside the system. Those inside any establishment can be habituated to the way things have always been done."[33]

These paragraphs barely touch the surface of this subject. Sexism must be viewed as an ethical challenge in medical education, because such bias can interfere with "seeing" and "hearing" patients and thus with establishing a therapeutic relationship. Stereotyping others always limits them, and given that gender bias is so prevalent in our society, medical educators should address this problem at all opportunities, for instance, during orientation, in classes on medical ethics and medical humanities, and in introduction to patient care classes. Open discussions of the dehumanizing effects of all forms of bias will encourage students to address problems as they arise and contribute to their development as empathic physicians. Any successful efforts to humanize medical education will improve the climate for students of both sexes and will result in more empathic care givers for patients.

Notes

1. Epigraph: C. Gilligan and S. Pollack, "The Vulnerable and Invulnerable Physician," in *Mapping the Moral Domain,* ed. C. Gilligan et al. (Cambridge, Mass.: Harvard University Press, 1988). Statistics from AAMC, *Women in Academic Medicine Statistics* (July 1993), table 1.

2. J. B. Miller, *Toward a New Psychology of Women,* 2nd ed. (Boston: Beacon Press, 1986).

3. All AAMC GQ refer to 1992 data.

4. American Association of University Women, *The AAUW Report: How Schools Shortchange Girls* (Washington, D.C.: AAUW, 1992).

5. K. H. Sheehan, D. V. Sheehan, K. White, A. Leibowitz, and D. C.

Baldwin, Jr., "A Pilot Study of Medical Student 'Abuse': Student Perceptions of Mistreatment and Misconduct in Medical School," *Journal of the American Medical Association*, 263:4 (1990):533–537.

6. J. A. Richman, J. A. Flaherty, K. M. Rospenda, and M. L. Christen, "Mental Health Consequences and Correlates of Reported Medical Student Abuse," *Journal of the American Medical Association*, 267:5 (1992):692–694, esp. 693.

7. W. C. Pauche and J. M. Miller, Jr., "Performances of Female Medical Students in an Obstetrics and Gynecology Clerkship," *Journal of Medical Education*, 61 (1986):323–325.

8. M. R. Inglehart and D. R. Brown, "Gender Differences in Values and Their Impact on Academic Achievement," paper presented at the tenth annual meeting of the International Society of Political Psychology, San Francisco, Calif., July 1987.

9. R. J. Paimes, L. J. Woodward, C. R. Blair, R. G. Roetzheim, and A. H. Herold, "The Influence on Students' Specialty Selections of Faculty Evaluations and Mini-Board Scores during Third-Year Clerkships," *Academic Medicine* 67:2 (February 1992):127–129.

10. P. J. Rutala et al., "The Influences of Student and Standardized Patient Genders on Scoring in an Objective Structured Clinical Examination," Supplement, *Academic Medicine* 66 (Sept. 1991):S28–30; J. A. Colliver, "The Interaction of Student Gender and Standardized-Patient Gender on Performance-Based Examination of Clinical Competence," Supplement, *Academic Medicine* 66 (September 1991):S31–33. Standardized patients are laypersons trained to simulate illnesses for purposes of medical student clinical training.

11. D. C. Baldwin et al., "Changes in Moral Reasoning during Medical School," Supplement, *Academic Medicine* 66 (September 1991):S1–3.

12. C. Gilligan, *In a Different Voice: Pychological Theory and Women's Development* (Cambridge, Mass.: Harvard University Press, 1982).

13. R. H. Coombs and H. C. Hovanessian, "Stress in the Role Constellation of Female Resident Physicians," *Journal of the American Medical Women's Association* 43:1 (January–February, 1988):23–27; M. T. Notman et al., "Stress and Adaptation in Medical Students: Who Is the Most Vulnerable?" *Comprehensive Psychiatry* 25 (1984):355–356.

14. L. R. Archer et al., "The Relationship between Residents' Characteristics, Their Street Experiences, and Their Psychosocial Adjustment at One Medical School," *Academic Medicine* 66 (1991):301–303.

15. L. J. Dickstein et al., "Psychiatric Impairment in Medical Students," *Academic Medicine* 65 (1990):588–593.

16. Gilligan and Pollack, "The Vulnerable," 261.

17. F. W. Hafferty, *Into the Valley: Death and the Socialization of Medical Students* (New Haven: Yale University Press, 1991), 200.

18. AMA Women in Medicine Project, *In the Marketplace*, 2nd ed. (Chicago: American Medical Association, 1987).

19. Personal communication from Charles Killian, Ph.D., Director, AAMC Student and Applicant Information Management System.

20. C. A. Bernstein et al., "Medical and Dental Students' Attitudes about the AIDS Epidemic," *Academic Medicine* 65 (1990):458–460.

21. B. Maheux et al., "Female Medical Practitioners: More Preventive and Patient Oriented?" *Medical Care* 28 (1990):87–92.

22. AAMC Faculty Roster, in AAMC, *Women in Academic Medicine Statistics* (July 1993), table 5.

23. Paimes et al., "The Influence," 127–129.

24. E. V. Calkins, T. L. Willoughby, and Louise M. Arnold, "Women Medical Students' Ratings of the Required Surgery Clerkship: Implications for Career Choice," *Journal of the American Medical Women's Association* 47:2 (March–April 1992):58–60.

25. J. Hadley, J. C. Cantor, R. J. Willke, J. Feder, and A. B. Cohen, "Young Physicians Most and Least Likely to Have Second Thoughts about a Career in Medicine," *Academic Medicine* 67:3 (March 1992):180–189.

26. Gilligan and Pollack, "The Vulnerable"; Hafferty, *Into the Valley*.

27. S. Lenhart and C. Evans, "Sexual Harassment and Gender Discrimination: A Primer for Women Physicians," *Journal of the American Medical Women's Association* 46 (1991):77–82.

28. C. Eisenberg, "Medicine Is No Longer a Man's Profession: Or, When the Men's Club Goes Coed It's Time to Change the Regulations," *New England Journal of Medicine* 321 (1989):1542–1544.

29. Hafferty, *Into the Valley*.

30. W. Levinson et al., "Women in Academic Medicine: Combining Career and Family," *New England Journal of Medicine* 321 (1989):1511–1517.

31. J. Bickel, *Medicine and Parenting: A Resource for Medical Students, Residents, Faculty, and Program Directors* (Washington, D.C.: Association of American Medical Colleges, 1991).

32. J. Bickel, *Building a Stronger Women's Program: Enhancing the Educational and Professional Environment* (Washington, D.C.: Association of American Medical Colleges, 1993).

33. S. Callahan, "Does Gender Make a Difference in Moral Decision Making?" *Second Opinion* (October 1991):67–77, esp. 74.

Notes on Contributors

RONALD ADELMAN, M.D., is an internist, geriatrician, and Chief of Geriatric Medicine at Winthrop University Hospital in Mineola, New York. His research interest is in the patient–physician relationship, particularly elderly patient–physician communication. Dr. Adelman has published in *The Gerontologist*, the *Journal of the American Geriatrics Society*, and *Aging and Society*.

STEPHEN J. BERGMAN, M.D., Ph.D., is Lecturer in Psychiatry at Harvard Medical School and Chairman of Clinical Projects at the Harvard Medical School, Division on Addictions. He is also an Affiliated Scholar at the Stone Center, Wellesley College. Under the pen name "Samuel Shem" he has published many novels and plays; his novel *The House of God* has been called "the best novel ever written about medical internship—a classic," and has sold over a million copies. He has been selected as one of the Boston Public Library's "Literary Lights," and as one of "Boston's Best Authors." With Janet Surrey, he is author of the play *Bill W. and Dr. Bob*, about the founding of Alcoholics Anonymous. He teaches a course for medical students on "how to stay human in medicine."

JANET BICKEL, M.A., is Assistant Vice-President for Women's Programs, Association of American Medical Colleges (AAMC). For the last eight years she has been working to improve the gender climate in medical schools and to promote the development of women leaders in academic medicine. She has spoken on gender-related issues at more than thirty medical schools and published articles on a broad spectrum of areas in academic medicine, including faculty tenure policies and student professional ethics. Previously, Ms. Bickel staffed AAMC's Organization of Student Representatives and Group on Student Affairs. She began her involvement with medical education at Brown University, where from 1972 to 1976 she served as admissions, financial aid, and student affairs officer for the new medical school.

LUCY M. CANDIB, M.D., is a family doctor who has taught and practiced family medicine, including obstetrics, in an urban neighborhood health center in Worcester, Massachusetts, for the past twenty years. A contributor to the first edition of *Our Bodies, Our Selves,* she has been an active participant in the women's health movement since medical school. Within the context of long-term doctor-patient relationships, she has put feminist principles to work in a multicultural setting. She has also focused attention on the concerns of women trainees and practitioners. She has lectured widely on the topics of sexual abuse and violence against women. In 1993 Dr. Candib was the co-recipient of the Society of Teachers of Family Medicine Award for Excellence in Education. She is the author of many articles and a forthcoming book on gender and medicine.

RITA CHARON, M.D., is a primary care internist and Associate Professor of Clinical Medicine at the College of Physicians and Surgeons of Columbia University. She is currently a doctoral candidate in the Department of English and Comparative Literature at Columbia University. A scholar in the field of literature and medicine, Dr. Charon teaches literature and narrative writing to medical students, house officers, and physicians. Her research interests include the narrative elements of doctor-patient interactions and linguistic examinations of doctor-patient discourse. She has published in *Literature and Medicine,* the *Annals of Internal Medicine, Soundings, Social Science & Medicine,* and the *Journal of Narrative and Life History.*

LORRAINE CODE, Ph.D., is Professor of Philosophy and Director of the Graduate Programme in Philosophy at York University in Toronto. In addition to numerous articles in philosophy and feminist theory, she is the author of *Epistemic Responsibility* (1987) and *What Can She Know? Feminist Theory and the Construction of Knowledge* (1991); and co-editor of *Feminist Perspectives: Philosophical Essays on Method and Morals* (1988) and *Changing Patterns: Women in Canada* (1988; 2nd ed., 1993). Her forthcoming book *Rhetorical Spaces: Essays on (Gendered) Locations* will be published by Routledge in 1995.

JULIA E. CONNELLY, M.D., is a general internist and Associate Professor of medicine at the University of Virginia who has practiced general medicine for ten years in a rural community near Charlottesville, Virginia. She is president-elect of the Society for Health and Human Values. The patient-physician relationship, the psychosocial aspects of health and illness, and the medical humanities, especially primary care ethics and literature, form the basis for her research and teaching. Currently her writing is focused on a collection of essays reflecting her experiences in medical practice.

MICHELE G. GREENE, D.P.H., is an Associate Professor in the Department of Health and Nutrition Sciences, Brooklyn College, City University of New York. She is also Senior Research Investigator, Division of Geriatrics, Winthrop-University Hospital, Mineola, New York. A social scientist, Dr. Greene has been conducting research on the physican-patient relationship for over fifteen years. In particular, she has studied the development, determinants, outcomes, and interactional dynamics of communication between primary care physicians and older patients. Her work has appeared in journals such as *Language and Communication, The Gerontologist,* and *Communication Research.*

PERRI KLASS, M.D., is a pediatrician at Dorchester House, a neighborhood health center in Boston, and Assistant Clinical Professor of Pediatrics at Boston University School of Medicine. She was graduated from Harvard Medical School in 1986, and did her residency in pediatrics at Children's Hospital in Boston, followed by a fellowship in Pediatric Infectious Diseases at Boston City Hospital. She has written extensively about medicine and medical training, including the books *Baby Doctor: A Pediatrician's Training,* and *A Not Entirely Benign Procedure: Four Years as a Medical Student,* as well as articles in publications ranging from the *New York Times* to *Glamour* to *Massachusetts Medicine.* She is also the author of the novels *Other Women's Children* and *Recombinations,* and a collection of short stories, *I Am Having an Adventure.* Her short fiction has won four O. Henry awards, and has been widely anthologized.

JOAN A. LANG, M.D., is Professor of Psychiatry and Behavioral Sciences, Director of Residency Training, and Coordinator of Educational Programs in the Department of Psychiatry and Behavioral Sciences at the University of Texas Medical Branch in Galveston. She teaches psychotherapy and psychoanalysis and is also Instructor at the Houston-Galveston Psychoanalytic Institute in Houston, Texas. Dr. Lang has co-edited the two-volume book *The Borderline Patient: Emerging Concepts in Diagnosis, Psychodynamics, and Treatment.* She is a member of the Committee of Women on Human Sexuality of the Group for the Advancement of Psychiatry and the Committee of Women of the Texas Society of Psychiatric Physicians. She is especially noted for her work concerning the feminine self and self psychology and treatment of women.

SUSAN E. LEDERER, Ph.D., is Associate Professor in the Department of Humanities at the Pennsylvania State University College of Medicine, where she teaches the history of American medicine and public health. Her research has focused on the history of medical experimentation involving human subjects—especially children and military personnel. She is currently at work on a history of animal experimentation in twentieth-century America.

MAUREEN A. MILLIGAN, Ph.D., is an Assistant Professor of Health Care Administration at the School of Allied Health Sciences at the University of Texas Medical Branch at Galveston. She received her Ph.D. in philosophy from Marquette University. Currently she is completing an M.A. in Medical Humanities at the Institute for the Medical Humanities and an M. P.AFF. at the Lyndon B. Johnson School of Public Affairs in Austin, Texas. Her areas of interest include health and welfare policy and ethics and addiction. Recent publications include "Reflections on Feminist Scepticism, the 'Maleness' of Philosophy and Postmodernism," in *Hypatia,* and book chapters on self-help and attitudinal healing, and the emergence of home health aides.

REGINA MORANTZ-SANCHEZ, Ph.D., teaches women's history and the history of medicine at the University of Michigan. She is editor of *In Her Own Words: Oral Histories of Women Physicians* (1982) and author of *Sympathy and Science: Women Physicians in American Medicine* (1985) and numerous articles on the history of women physicians. She is presently working on a third book that uses a spectacular nineteenth-century libel trial between a woman surgeon and the Brooklyn *Eagle* newspaper to explore themes involving professionalization, gender, and the emergence of gynecological surgery in nineteenth-century America.

ELLEN SINGER MORE, Ph.D., is Associate Professor of History of Medicine and Medical Humanities at the Institute for the Medical Humanities, University of Texas Medical Branch at Galveston, where she teaches the history of medicine, medical humanities, gender and professionalism, and the ethics of scientific research. In addition, she acts as a consultant to faculty and nurses in the departments of Obstetrics-Gynecology, Pediatrics, Psychiatry, and Surgery on issues of professional ethics. Her publications include numerous articles on the history of women physicians in American medicine and a forthcoming book, *Restoring the Balance: Women Physicians and the Profession of Medicine* (Harvard).

CAROL C. NADELSON, M.D., is currently Editor-in-Chief of American Psychiatric Press, Professor of Psychiatry at Tufts University School of Medicine, Lecturer on Psychiatry at Harvard Medical School, and is on the staff of The Cambridge Hospital. She is a past president of the American Psychiatric Association, and was formerly a Fellow at the Center for Advanced Study in the Behavioral Sciences. She is the author of almost two hundred publications and co-editor of thirteen books. Dr. Nadelson is a frequent lecturer on medical ethics, medical and psychiatric education, women's health, the psychology of women, gender issues in medicine, and other topics in psychiatry.

MARIAN GRAY SECUNDY, Ph.D., is Professor and Director of the Program in Medical Ethics at Howard University College of Medicine. She has been a Visiting Scholar at the University of San Francisco Health Policy Institute, the University of Chicago's Pritzker School of Medicine, the National Leadership Training Program in Clinical Medical Ethics, Michigan State University, and Hiram College. A practicing psychotherapist, Dr. Secundy is also editor of *Trials, Tribulations, and Celebrations: African-American Perspectives on Health, Illness, Aging, and Loss.* She served in 1993 as co-chair of the Ethics Working Group of Hillary Rodham Clinton's Health Care Task Force.

JANET L. SURREY, Ph.D., is a clinical psychologist and Clinical Instructor in Psychology at Harvard Medical School. She is a founding member of the Women's Program at McLean Hospital, and in her capacity as Research Associate at the Stone Center, Wellesley College, she has published numerous papers and has become noted internationally for her work on theories of women's psychological development. She is co-author of *Women's Growth in Connection: Writings from the Stone Center.* As Adjunct Professor at the Episcopal Divinity School in Cambridge, Massachusetts, she has taught and written on spirituality and addiction. With Dr. Bergman she is co-director of The Center for Gender Relations, in Boston.

Index